Managing Managed Care

A Mental Health Practitioner's
Survival Guide

Managing Managed Care

A Mental Health Practitioner's Survival Guide

by

Michael Goodman, M.D.
Janet Brown, R.N., B.S.M.C., C.P.H.Q.
Pamela Deitz, L.C.S.W., M.F.C.C.

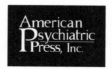

American Psychiatric Press, Inc.

Washington, DC
London, England

Note: The authors have worked to ensure that all information in this book concerning drug dosages, schedules, and routes of administration is accurate as of the time of publication and consistent with standards set by the U.S. Food and Drug Administration and the general medical community. As medical research and practice advance, however, therapeutic standards may change. For this reason and because human and mechanical errors sometimes occur, we recommend that readers follow the advice of a physician who is directly involved in their care or the care of a member of their family.

Books published by the American Psychiatric Press, Inc., represent the views and opinions of the individual authors and do not necessarily represent the policies and opinions of the Press or the American Psychiatric Association.

Copyright © 1992 American Psychiatric Press, Inc.
ALL RIGHTS RESERVED
Manufactured in the United States of America on
acid-free paper.
95 94 93 92 4 3 2 1
First Edition

American Psychiatric Press, Inc.
1400 K Street, N.W.
Washington, DC 20005

Library of Congress Cataloging-in-Publication Data

Goodman, Michael, 1945–
  Managing managed care : a mental health practitioner's survival guide. / by Michael Goodman, Janet Brown, Pamela Deitz — 1st ed.
    p.   cm.
  Includes bibliographical references and index.
  ISBN 0-88048-369-5 (alk. paper)
  1. Psychiatric disability evaluation. 2. Managed care plans (Medical care). I. Brown, Janet, 1945– . II. Deitz, Pamela, 1949– . III. Title.
  [DNLM: 1. Documentation—methods. 2. Managed Care Programs—organization & administration. 3. Mental Health Services—organization & administration. 4. Quality of Health Care. WM 30 G653m]
RC470.G66 1992
362.2'068—dc20
DNLM/DLC   92-7051
for Library of Congress   CIP

British Library Cataloguing in Publication Data

A CIP record is available from the British Library.

To our parents—who encouraged us
to question and learn;
and
to our colleagues and patients—
who continue to teach us.

Contents

About the Authors

Michael Goodman, M.D. is a clinical psychiatrist in private practice in Beverly Hills and Pasadena, California. He attended Tufts Medical School and completed his psychiatry residency at Northwestern University in Chicago. Dr. Goodman has 10 years experience as a physician advisor with the former California PSRO and its current successor, California Medical Review, Inc., and consults with psychiatric hospitals and mental health facilities on quality improvement, utilization management, and corroborative documentation formats for same. He is also a clinical faculty member of the UCLA School of Medicine, Department of Psychiatry and Biobehavioral Sciences.

Janet A. Brown, R.N., B.S.M.C., C.P.H.Q., is a consultant in quality, utilization, and risk management with psychiatric and medical-surgical, acute and ambulatory, healthcare organizations. She has 14 years of experience in the evaluation, development, and implementation of effective systems and programs that meet federal and state regulations, voluntary accreditation standards, and external review requirements in healthcare. Janet is the author of *The Quality Management Professional's Study Guide,* 7th Edition, and serves as instructor for quality management professionals preparing for the certification exam. She has also chaired the national Healthcare Quality Educational Foundation.

Pamela M. Deitz, L.C.S.W., M.F.C.C., is a psychotherapist in private practice. A graduate of the University of Southern California, Ms. Deitz has continued to work in both agency and hospital settings. Her recent role as developer and clinical director of an adolescent treatment program heightened her awareness of and interest in the impact of managed care on all clinical disciplines providing mental health services.

Acknowledgments

We wish to express our gratitude to a number of people without whom this book would never have been written, at least not in its present form.

Our initial ideas for this book were germinating in isolation, and, to that end, we wish to thank the entire treatment staff at Ingleside Hospital and the adolescent treatment team at Terrace Plaza Hospital for their receptivity to "planting" our seedling notions in their treatment planning sessions and medical record documentation formats. Both of these staffs patiently tolerated one hybrid of our system after another, until we were finally able to "get it right," and we are indebted to them. A special thanks goes to Othea Byers, who provided the moral support while we all struggled with these numerous modifications.

We appreciate the time and earnestness of David Kater, Ph.D., Steve Hayes, M.D., and Jeanne Schaffer, R.N.C., who reviewed the clinical content of our system and offered valuable suggestions. We thank Neil Andrews, M.D., Director of Behavioral Health Access, Blue Cross of California; and Lucy Anderson, Director of Provider Systems, and Lester Goldstein, M.D., Medical Director, both of Preferred Health Care, Ltd.—West, for their original ideas on improving the structure of our system to most effectively meet the information requirements of external review and managed care organizations. James Grotstein, M.D., will readily recognize many of his ideas permeating our theoretical and clinical understanding of patients and their care. We are pleased to assert that psychoanalysis and managed care may not be as estranged as they appear to be.

We had the good fortune of finding in Carol Nadelson, M.D., an editor who delicately guided us through the heated controversy between managed care and mental health during the early phases of the manuscript review process. She delicately tamed our initial fervor while still preserving the original meaning and intent of this book.

We thank our patients for persevering with us in the struggle to understand the vicissitudes of managed care and its impact on the quality and accessibility of mental health treatment. Please note that we have changed the names and identifying information of the individuals in the case studies extensively so that the privacy of these individuals is protected. In some cases a composite was created from several persons in order to protect their anonymity. If the names of persons or clinical presentations in this book bear any resemblance to those actual persons, the similarity is purely accidental.

Reserving our most important acknowledgment for last, we wish to thank our families, who never failed to support us while tolerating countless meetings, interminable telephone discussions, and a seemingly endless number of revisions and rewrites. Their patience and loyalty are commendable. We must give special thanks on behalf of Janet to Warren Brown, Ph.D., for a husband's patience, a brain researcher's scrutiny, and an innovator's ideas for future applications of the method and system presented in this book.

M.G.
J.B.
P.D.

Preface

Healthcare providers are under seige by insurers, employers, and government to control spiraling costs, improve access to services, minimize risk, and, at the same time, provide quality care. As an outgrowth of this mandate to "do more with less," providers are now encountering a multiplicity of new and unprecedented external review mechanisms for managing patient care and the healthcare dollar. Managed care is a fact, not a fad, and this places an unanticipated, perhaps unwelcome, imperative on healthcare practitioners to understand the external review process in order to effectively respond to it.

The management of mental health services presents a particularly acute problem for both the practitioners and the external reviewers. Mental healthcare is a multidisciplinary and, therefore, multilingual field. Add to this the growing and diverse demands of various managed care organizations and third-party payers, and the potential for communication difficulties is compounded. This frustrating situation was the impetus for the authors to write this book. When we met, we were coming from very different perspectives. A collision was unavoidable.

Pamela Deitz, the program director for an inpatient adolescent unit, was seeking consultation on how to develop a new quality and utilization management program prior to the unit's first accreditation survey; Janet Brown, the quality management consultant, was experiencing a great deal of difficulty in evaluating the quality and appropriateness of care in that program based on the documentation she found in the medical records; and Dr. Michael Goodman, the psychiatric director of the program, was feeling increasingly frustrated with his efforts in communicating the necessity of additional hospitalization for his patients to several new external review organizations. We quickly discovered that we were each operating by our own and very different sets of "rules." Each of us was employing some terminology unfamiliar to the others, and we were often using terms that, in fact, we neither consensually agreed upon nor understood in the same way. That was 8 years ago.

We became convinced that there must be a better way to document all aspects of mental healthcare treatment and to communicate with those individuals, groups, and agencies who now need and have the right to know about the treatment. We decided to develop a meaningful, serviceable language of treatment and a documentation system for all mental health professionals who provide direct patient care and whose treatment services may be subject to review prior to reimbursement. These practitioners include psychiatrists, clinical psychologists, clinical social workers, and, in those states that provide the licensure or certification, marriage, family, and child therapists.

Our aim in this book is to provide all mental health professionals, regardless of their level of training or clinical orientation, with an easy-to-learn, easy-to-use system for communicating with external reviewers and documenting the quality of care. This book is also written for the students of mental health disciplines and their clinical supervisors to prepare the prospective practitioner for responding effectively to these new accountability and reimbursement realities.

Our method for documenting and communicating the necessity, appropriateness, and effectiveness of mental healthcare services is the common avenue upon which the practitioner, the external reviewer, and the quality management professional can communicate and travel in amicable parallel. In our experience with external review organizations, this system smooths out what has heretofore often been a bumpy ride for mental health professionals. While the final destinations of mental healthcare and external review in this country are still largely unknown, we hope that this guide will help practitioners avoid collisions with reviewers and ensure each other's survival.

Chapter 1

Introduction

Just being a competent therapist today is not enough to keep one in his or her job. If the title of this book has at all enticed or intrigued you, it is because of your awareness of the increasing demands being made upon mental health professionals to convey information about patients and their treatment services to reviewers who want to know about them. Having to justify one's treatment services in order to remain in business is one of the most delicate and fiercely debated issues in mental health today. Diametrically opposed professional, political, economic, social, and ethical points of view, coupled with a conspicuous absence of semantic consistency regarding such concepts as "quality care," will no doubt perpetuate this complex controversy into the foreseeable future.

We, the authors, have made a deliberate effort to avoid entering into this heated fray. It is not our intent to take sides in the controversy or assign any blame. What we hope to do in this book is 1) clarify for the reader the issues of practitioner accountability as they relate to both reimbursement decisions and quality monitoring, and 2) introduce an effective proactive response to a current reality that according to all predictions is not going to go away.

Why Is This Book a "Survival Guide"?

In a crisis, continuing to exist becomes the first priority. The evidence is now in that the American healthcare system is indeed in a crisis. Healthcare in the United States is the most expensive in the world, and yet life expectancy is shorter than in 15 other countries, and infant mortality is worse than in 22 other countries (Hilts 1991). Healthcare expenditures in the United States have surged from less than 6% of the national domestic spending in 1965 to more than 12% today, and it is estimated that by the year 2000, healthcare costs will consume at least 15% of the nation's total output of goods and services (Gray 1991).

The tension in the private sector is particularly acute. Businesses are now watching their healthcare spending devour ever larger portions of their profits. In the 1960s, businesses spent about 4 to 8 cents of each dollar of profit on healthcare. In 1990, it was up to 50 cents per dollar, and it is expected to reach 60 cents by the year 2000 (Hilts 1991).

The increase in costs for mental healthcare services in particular is even more staggering. In 1980, the total cost for mental health and chemical dependency treatment was $35 billion. These costs spiraled to $50 billion in 1983 and to over $80 billion in 1990 (Kessler 1989). Although just 3% of the population uses psychiatric insurance benefits, psychiatric treatment accounted for 25% of all hospital days in 1987 and 30% in 1988 (Kessler 1989).

A precipitous slashing of coverage for mental healthcare services, and, in some cases, the elimination of mental health benefits altogether, were unfortunate early responses by a number of employers and insurers to these rapidly escalating costs. But even with such radical measures, the spiral of spending has shown little or no sign of significantly abating. This underscores the urgency with which government and big business are seeking new ways to contain healthcare costs and spend healthcare dollars more effectively. As the trustees of the Social Security Board in their annual report on the health of Medicare and Social Security stated, "Reducing costs needs to be continued in close combination with mechanisms that will assure that the quality of healthcare is not adversely affected" (Rosenblatt 1991).

Managed care is growing by leaps and bounds, not because mental health professionals and patients have fallen in love with it, but because employers, who have become dissatisfied with the skyrocketing costs of fee-for-service care, are hopeful that the promise of predicted savings through management of the care can be achieved. In the midst of this crisis, mental health professionals are increasingly finding themselves having to justify the necessity for, and demonstrate the quality of, their services.

Most clinical training programs for mental health professionals currently do not systematically train their students on how to survive this crisis and meet the demand for increased accountability. The Chinese calligraphy for the word "crisis" is a combination of two Chinese characters: "catastrophe" and "opportunity." In the face of this impending catastrophe, we took the opportunity to develop some "survival tools" for those who are most dearly affected by this current crisis in healthcare.

What Is "Managed Care"?

The term "managed care" has unfortunately been diluted and misused, and there is no longer consensual agreement on the meaning of this term. In its broadest definition, managed care is any patient care that is not determined solely by the provider. "External review" is a general term for any outside group or organization that examines or scrutinizes healthcare treatment services. Some external review organizations call themselves managed care or case management groups when, in fact, the only aspect of quality care that appears to be managed is the immediate expense, at times without any consideration of possible long-range costs, quality, or risk. There are other managed care organizations that do undertake the total management of the patient's care, from wellness through chronic illness. Some of these "health management" or "preferred provider" organizations utilize vertically integrated systems of care delivery that allow patients to traverse a variety of levels of care (e.g., hospitalization, residential treatment, day treatment, intensive outpatient therapy, medication management, etc.).

In *The Profit Motive and Patient Care,* Bradford H. Gray comments that for the time being, we are living through "an unplanned national experiment to see how much medical care can be managed through the use of incentives and review mechanisms" (Gray 1991, p. 262). Our book is intended to help the mental health professional cope with these "external" review mechanisms, including managed care. Providing incentives to practitioners to discount their fees and join preferred provider organizations (PPOs) or health maintenance organizations (HMOs)—in return for such perquisites as increased patient referrals and prompt reimbursement—is another form of medical care management that will not be addressed here. How to make one's way through the maze of myriad PPO networks and HMOs is the subject of another book that needs to be written.

Why the Term
"Mental Healthcare Practitioner"?

A number of the same-coded treatment procedures in mental healthcare are performed by psychiatrists, clinical psychologists, clinical social workers, and marriage, family, and child therapists. All of these disciplines are being monitored for the quality of their services in inpatient settings, and all are likely to have their services reviewed prior to reimbursement. Which discipline is in fact the most appropriate to deliver which treatment services is a question yet to be decisively answered.

Also, organizations managing mental healthcare benefits utilize a variety of mental healthcare disciplines to provide different treatment services, from initial evaluations and crisis intervention to long-term individual psychotherapy; HMOs do not always provide for a psychiatric evaluation except under certain conditions. This book does not "take a stand" on these practices that may or may not affect the quality of the care being given. Nonetheless, because all providers of services, regardless of their discipline, are required to justify the necessity for, and document the quality of, their treatments, this book is written for all mental health practitioners.

Chapters 2 and 3 of this book detail the historical development of managed care, external, and quality review. The remaining chapters take the practitioner step by step through the external review process and introduce a method for responding to the various questions posed by external reviewers. The system we propose is by no means perfect and is not meant to be the final word in treatment documentation. However, having shared this material with three of the largest nationally based organizations that manage mental healthcare benefits exclusively, we were pleased to note that the documentation-communication model proposed in this book conforms with and meets their information requirements for making medical necessity and appropriateness determinations.

That this current state of affairs may be quite irritating to the busy practitioner who wishes to devote more time to direct patient care, we do not disagree. At the same time, we have decided to follow the lead of the oyster, which, "when irritated by a grain of sand, makes a pearl." We hope that this book contains some pearls that will help you, the practitioner, survive the external review process a bit more comfortably and with slightly less irritation.

Chapter 2

The Public Demand for Practitioner Accountability

"Your services are subject to continued review."

Prior to the first federally mandated professional standards review organization (PSRO) in 1972, the primary responsibilities of healthcare providers were to diagnose, to treat, and, above all, primum non nocere *(to do no harm). In this chapter we survey the broadening of the healthcare practitioner's duties from private responsibility to public accountability. With the implementation of the PSROs, accountability for utilization of healthcare services became a requirement for reimbursement. The Peer Review Improvement Act of 1982 mandated both utilization and quality review and, for the first time, required Medicare providers to release patient information to a PSRO for private review. Private payers could now initiate review prior to payment—hence the feverish proliferation of external review organizations, managed care businesses, and case management companies. These organizations all ask questions now about the medical necessity and quality of healthcare services—questions that most mental health professionals have never been trained to answer.*

The Babylonians were among the first people to develop a systematic practice of healthcare. Their writings as far back as 1600 B.C. include instructions for specific recipes of herbs to treat certain conditions. Occasionally, treatment was overseen or administered by magicians who might also drive out the demons responsible for the afflictions being treated. It was to be another 11 centuries, however, before the quality of healthcare was identified to be the designated responsibility of its practitioners. An oath of physician responsibility attributed to Hippocrates in the 5th century B.C. states:

> I swear by Apollo, the physician, that according to my ability and judgment . . . I will follow that method of treatment which I consider for the benefit of my patients, and abstain from whatever is deleterious and mischievous. Whatever in connection with my professional practice or not in connection with it, I may see or hear in the lives of men, which ought not be spoken abroad, I will not divulge . . . (Lyon and Petricelli 1978)

For the following 24 centuries, practitioner accountability for the quality of healthcare services was understood and accepted as the practitioner's internal professional sense of moral and ethical responsibility. The established duties of healthcare providers were to diagnose, treat, and, above all, "do no harm" (an axiom attributed to the Hippocratic oath but in fact coming from another Hippocratic work, "Epidemics").

Within the last 25 years, however, the responsibility for the quality of healthcare services has been significantly redefined for practitioners and, in fact, has been considerably expanded. As a result, today's healthcare practitioners are finding an alarming number of work hours consumed by the demands of internal and external utilization and quality review—hours that in the past had been available for direct patient care. How this came to be is a tale of the transformation of medical care and medical information from "private practice" to the public domain.

The first half of the 20th century witnessed initial efforts on the part of healthcare practitioners to monitor internally the quality of their own peers. In 1910, Dr. Abraham Flexner released a study of the quality of medical schools in the United States that stimulated the elimination of "diploma mills." Three years later, the American College of Surgeons was formed as an accrediting body, generating operational standards for medical education and performance. Simultaneously, internal monitoring of healthcare practices was gradually undertaken by state licensing boards and the various city, regional, state, and national medical associations or societies to which healthcare practitioners typically belonged. State licensing boards and medical associations, however, have been characteristically reactive—that is, investigating legal actions taken elsewhere or complaints made by others directly to them concerning a particular practitioner.

In 1952, the Joint Commission on Accreditation of Hospitals—now the Joint Commission on Accreditation of Healthcare Organizations (Joint Commission)—succeeded the American College of Surgeons as the responsible organization for monitoring compliance with defined operational standards. Since then, the notion that healthcare practitioners are individually and internally responsible and internally accountable for the quality of patient care has been challenged and subsequently redefined. The precedent for institutional liability for the quality of medical care provided by physicians was expanded in the 1965 judicial decision *Darling v. Charleston Community Memorial Hospital.*

In 1972, amendments to the Social Security Act mandated the establishment of professional standards review organizations (PSROs), heralding a new level of external professional accountability for the cost, quality, and appropriateness of healthcare services (Social Security Amendments 1972).

In hospital settings, the quality assurance department had originally functioned only peripherally to maintain Joint Commission accreditation. In the 1982 judicial decision *Elam v. College Park Hospital,* the ultimate legal and fiduciary responsibility for the quality of healthcare was placed upon the governing body. As a result, *quality improvement*—a term that has replaced quality assurance and more clearly communicates the purpose of such activities—moved from the basement into the boardroom. Also in 1982, the Peer Review Improvement Act replaced the PSRO program with the new *utilization and quality control peer review organization* (now shortened to PRO) and for the first time required Medicare providers to release patient information to a PSRO or PRO for private review. After this pivotal piece of legislation, the door was opened for private payers as well to initiate review prior to payment. The result was a feverish proliferation of external review organizations, managed care businesses, and case management companies, all of which were asking questions about the medical necessity and quality of healthcare services. Depending on the answers they received, these external reviewers and third-party payers had now been given the legal right to significantly reduce or totally deny reimbursement for those services.

The breadth of practitioner accountability has continued to expand since the implementation of the Medicare Prospective Payment System (PPS) (Title VI of the Social Security Amendments) in 1983. The PPS utilizes the patient classification system of diagnosis-related groups (DRGs) originally devised by John Thompson and Robert Fetter at Yale in 1975 (Fetter 1980). The DRGs classify patients into at least 475 categories based on diagnoses, procedures (e.g., surgery), and comorbid conditions. The PPS replaced the charge-based retrospective payment system for all but a few classes of hospitals. Among those exemptions were psychiatric and alcohol and other drug abuse treatment hospitals and, on application, psychiatric and alcohol abuse units in general hospitals (U.S. Department of Health and Human Services 1983).

At about the same time, and in response to spiraling costs and concern for the efficacy and the medical necessity of mental healthcare services in general, many private insurers began to significantly reduce available benefits for psychiatric and chemical dependency services. More recently, employers have begun to opt for health insurance from those third-party payers that incorporate a "managed care" approach to mental healthcare and chemical dependency treatment. As a result of these developments, mental healthcare practitioners have now come to find themselves evermore pressed to respond to questions posed by a medically sophisticated and financially savvy consumer-payer public that wants to know about the quality and cost of healthcare services being purchased.

It is now a prevailing belief that medical knowledge and the activities of its practitioners belong to the community. To this end, a national data bank designed to capture aberrant practices and behaviors of physicians, dentists, and osteopaths was congressionally mandated in 1986 (Healthcare Quality Improvement Act). The Medicare and Medicaid Patient and Program Protection Act of 1987 expanded the reporting requirements to include podiatrists, clinical psychologists, and essentially any other licensed independent practitioner. This data bank, operated by UNISYS Corporation under contract with the U.S. Public Health Service (PHS), began operating on September 1, 1990, and is a computerized compilation of disciplinary actions and malpractice payouts against independent practitioners nationwide. The PHS states that "entities that provide healthcare services and conduct formal peer review to improve quality will be obliged to report disciplinary actions to the bank and are entitled to receive data from it." Such entities are defined to include state- and federally recognized health maintenance organizations (HMOs) and group or prepaid medical practices. Hospitals, state medical licensing boards, professional societies that do peer review, liability insurers, and individuals and their attorneys have data bank reporting and querying responsibilities and rights.

Further, the Joint Commission is now actively involved in the development of "clinical indicators" (Joint Commission 1990b). These measures are specialty-specific standards of care with defined thresholds of acceptability based upon patient outcome. The Joint Commission plans to have on-line access to this set of clinical (as well as other organizational, financial, and administrative) data to facilitate ongoing, concurrent monitoring and evaluation of the quality of healthcare. A 10-year schedule is projected for the medical specialties, and it is to be divided into three phases: 1) obstetrics and anesthesia (Phase 1); 2) cardiovascular, oncology, and acute trauma (Phase 2); and surgery, mental health, and long-term care (Phase 3).

Thus, as healthcare and the documentation of healthcare services continue to "go public," so too do the behavior and thought processes of its providers. The once-held belief that "healthcare is healthcare is healthcare" has been dispelled as a "Merlin's myth," challenged by consumers and payers whose faith in the uniform quality of healthcare has been eroding and corroding over time. "Private practice" is becoming an endangered species. Unless mental healthcare practitioners can articulate what they are doing for their patients and also convincingly explain why they are doing it, purchasers and providers are going to be increasingly unwilling to pay for their services. If mental healthcare services are too subjective to quantify, they "may well be too subjective to pay for" (Brown 1991).

Mental healthcare providers must understand what external reviewers need to know, and they must have a means of communicating their response so that their services can be reimbursed. The intention of reviewers is not to doubt the clinicians' expertise or their capacity to make good clinical decisions. External reviewers want to know *why* treatment decisions are made. Practitioners are being asked to articulate their clinical rationale for the recommended treatment, and, for the first time, to provide the supportive, convincing clinical evidence that is the basis for that treatment decision—what is known as "articulating the process of care." Clinicians are not systematically educated about the value of articulating and documenting their own (usually intuitively accurate and preconscious) thought processes. Instead, they are trained to make the expedient, though tunneled, leap from diagnosis to treatment (as articulated by Hippocrates circa 500 B.C.) with nary a glance into the chasm of treatment choices and alternative care options that have become the focus of today's external reviewers.

External review at present is often experienced by the clinician as an intrusion—an invasion by an inquisitor-reviewer who challenges not only the practitioner's authority but also his or her historical right to operate in private.[1] In fact, external review is a request for information that will justify what the clinician already knows to be true. It is not necessarily the treatment decision that is being questioned. Rather, it is the expert's clinical rationale for that decision that is being examined. Mental healthcare practitioners who are tradition-

---

[1]This conflict is made explicit in the title of a 1982 article that appeared in the *American Journal of Psychiatry*: "Psychotherapy Research Evidence and Reimbursement Decisions: Bambi Meets Godzilla" (Parloff 1982).

ally trained to ask questions to explain the thinking, motives, and behavior of others are now finding themselves being asked to explain their own thinking and motives in treating their patients.

External review has become an increasingly cumbersome and time-consuming onus on the mental healthcare practitioner. The language of *impairments* introduced in this book was developed to alleviate this burden. It will be repeated throughout the book that impairment terminology is a behavioral language of treatment and is not meant to compete or conflict with DSM-III-R diagnostic nomenclature. (More will be said about this in Chapter 4.) Dialogue with quality management consultants, third-party payers, and managed care organizations confirms the dire necessity for terse, objective, behavioral descriptors of psychiatric patients and the care they receive. Although this insistence on objectification and quantification may offend the sensibilities of those dedicated to the art (and perhaps mystery) of mental healthcare, the posture of the payers appears to be this: If the clinical necessity and outcomes of mental healthcare services are too subjective to measure and quantify, then they may well be too subjective to pay for.

Two decades ago, Lawrence Weed (1969) prophesied that "the economic and organizational aspects of medical care, to a far greater degree than students are presently aware, will determine the quality and quantity of care they will be able to deliver" (p. 122). We are now there. The purpose of this book is therefore twofold: 1) to clarify for the mental healthcare professional what reviewers need to know, and 2) to introduce a behavioral language of treatment and a method for effectively and efficiently responding to external reviewers and accreditation organizations, and to nationwide concerns for quality and value of, and access to, the healthcare product.

Chapter 3

The Need for a Common Behavioral Language of Treatment

"Are your services medically necessary?"

There is a diversity of mental healthcare services and an equally diverse, variously trained admixture of external reviewers. Current methods of treatment documentation do not effectively communicate the clinical rationale for mental healthcare services and the patient's progress as a result of treatment. The omnipresent "patient problem list" is inadequate for communicating what reviewers need to know before authorizing reimbursement for services. This situation argues for a common language of readily understood patient behavioral dysfunctions.

External review for the clinical necessity of mental healthcare services historically began at the hospital level and then only after treatment was well underway or completed. In the mid-1970s, "external review" of patients receiving inpatient psychiatric or chemical dependency services took the form of the "request for additional information" letters to the practitioner or retrospective chart review. In 1988, only five million people with indemnity insurance had their mental healthcare reviewed by case managers. It is estimated that by 1993 that number will increase to 50 million, and less than 20% of the population will have traditional indemnity insurance without any element of managed care (Kessler 1989).

In our experience in Southern California, more than 80% of private psychiatric inpatients now require certification or authorization for hospital services prior to admission, and their cases are then concurrently reviewed for medical necessity at least weekly. Preauthorization and concurrent review for outpatient mental healthcare services are becoming increasingly common as accountability expands from the inpatient facility to practitioners' offices. Quality of care is now being assessed by insurers, employers, managed care organizations, external review organizations, and accrediting agencies. The knowledge that this monitoring is occurring and that it is directly linked to reimbursement for treatment services has indeed succeeded in getting the practitioners' attention.

Disturbingly, the individuals and agencies charged with obtaining this information represent multifariously vested, diverse interest groups. Further, the reviewers themselves possess widely varied (and in some cases no) mental health clinical backgrounds. To complicate the problem, third-party payers and managed care organizations approach mental healthcare providers with far from uniform standards for what constitutes quality treatment of mental and substance abuse disorders. At the same time, the responsibility and accountability for the quality of mental healthcare services have been extended and redefined by the Joint Commission to include all the disciplines that may treat mental disorders primarily and/or have an impact on their care secondarily. This, of course, includes any billable or potentially billable mental healthcare service.

It is inevitable that before long *all* providers of mental healthcare services at *all* levels of service intensity (i.e., inpatient, partial hospitalization, residential treatment, and outpatient) will be required to document and communicate the process and quality of their care. As mentioned earlier, the Joint Commission is continually sharpening its focus and expanding and redefining its parameters in monitoring and evaluating quality in mental healthcare in acute inpatient and residential treatment settings. The collective monitoring and evaluation of the quality of each treatment modality (i.e., each potentially billable service) measures the overall quality of clinical care a patient receives.

In response to this broadening of responsibility for the quality of mental healthcare services, we have chosen to define the clinical components of patient care by treatment modality (e.g., individual psychotherapy) rather than by treatment discipline (e.g., psychiatrist, psychologist, social worker). The modalities utilized on a psychiatric inpatient service providing comprehensive multidisciplinary treatment might include, but certainly are not limited to, the following:

✳ Individual psychotherapy
✳ Psychopharmacotherapy
✳ Electroconvulsive therapy
✳ Nursing
✳ Discharge planning services
✳ Individual family therapy
✳ Multiple family therapy
✳ Group psychotherapy
✳ Occupational therapy
✳ Recreational therapy
✳ Creative arts therapy (e.g., psychodrama)
✳ Physical therapy
✳ Biofeedback therapy
✳ Substance abuse counseling
✳ Nutritional and dietary counseling
✳ Educational services

The confusion between quality of care, cost of care, standards of care, and justification for care understandably creates a baffling state of affairs for the mental healthcare practitioner—in large part because there is still considerable debate as to just what constitutes quality mental healthcare services in particular and how one defines quality healthcare in general! Practitioners have been trained and are largely still trained to provide "high quality" care—that is, care that offers available services within accepted standards, utilizing all state-of-the-art technologies and generating clinical data from that care to make further scientific advances in the treatment of disease. Also, high-quality care has been the traditional expectation, requirement, and often the demand of the buyer of healthcare services. As recently as the mid 1970s, quality healthcare was based on two precepts—"Doctor knows best" and "Spend whatever it takes"—the cost of which is now prohibitive. The increasing elderly population, the constant (and increasingly expensive) technological progress, the public demand for quality (and concomitant expensive malpractice settlements), and the fierce competition for the healthcare dollar (advertising) are guaranteed to propel healthcare costs yet higher.

In order to monitor and evaluate the quality of patient care, one must examine a number of aspects of the care:

1. Is the care *appropriate* (i.e., clinically necessary) for the condition?
2. Is the provider *competent* to provide that care?
3. Is the care *effective*?
4. Is the care *cost-efficient*?
5. Is the care *accessible*?
6. Is the care *safe*?
7. Is the *patient satisfied*?

These are questions that mental healthcare practitioners may have never asked or been asked before.

When faced with an external review, the practitioner currently has no idea which of these parameters of quality monitoring are being addressed. For example, a growing number of large employers are asking health insurers and prepaid healthcare plans to come up with numbers that measure not only costs but also the quality of the care based upon patient outcome. One corporation with 66,700 employees plans to evaluate the quality of healthcare services of six health maintenance organizations (HMOs) with which it recently signed contracts and will continue to do so based upon whether or not the patients say that they are satisfied with their treatment. A Rand Corporation study (unpublished data, 1989) currently in progress has determined that patient satisfaction—the subjective report of how much better patients are feeling after treatment—is as valid a predictor of the quality of the care they have received as either a post-treatment physical examination or the cost. Responses to questionnaires distributed to patients during and after treatment may turn out to be the most accurate predictor of the competence and effectiveness of the services the patients received (Rand Corporation, unpublished data, 1989).

A common language of clinical data elements that is readily understood by all parties concerned is desperately needed. Ideally, this is a language that is useful in documenting the progress of treatment in the medical record as well as one that communicates the thought processes (clinical rationales) of the treater. This language must be easily understood and interpretable both by the professionals with multiple levels of clinical expertise who are documenting the treatment and by the equally diverse external reviewers who use that information to make reimbursement determinations. Current documentation methods for mental healthcare services are inadequate for this task. And the fact that several disciplines may perform similar services (e.g., individual psychotherapy) is an additional source of confusion for the external reviewer and again suggests that documentation of treatment components be divided by modality rather than by clinical discipline.

The difficulty in extrapolating from the medical record what treatment is being implemented for a patient and why it is being utilized is not a new concern. In 1969, Lawrence Weed commented that "at present no operational system exists that permits a medical teacher or member of an accrediting agency to take a patient's record . . . and assess whether current medical standards are being properly applied" (p. 122). Loosely structured and organized by diagnosis, the medical records of Weed's day were observed to be "simply static, pro forma repositories of medical observations and activities grouped in the meaningless order of source—whether doctor or nurse, laboratory or X-ray department" (p. vii). It was in reaction to this arcane and archaic method of collecting, organizing, and recording patient care data that the problem-oriented record was conceived and promulgated.

The "Weed system" was introduced as a documentation system that provided practitioners with a mechanism for not only documenting the reasons (problems) for initiating patient care but also, and more importantly, for graphically displaying the decision-making processes that determined the progress of that care. This system was designed to facilitate ready access to patient care data for meaningful treatment planning and concurrent case review, as well as to expedite retrieval of data for retrospective research and education. The patient "problem list" and the "subjective-objective-assessment-plan" (SOAP) format were conceived as operational mechanisms for ensuring and expanding the usefulness of the patient record. The patient problem list was to be the dynamic reflection of the evolving thought process of the practitioner as well as a means of tracking the clinical progress of the patient.

When psychiatry seized the problem-oriented record and applied it to psychiatric inpatient care, the essential dynamism of the Weed system was either lost or abandoned. The "patient problems" currently found in psychiatric records appear to be no more than landings upon which the treatment team rests rather than stairs that are used to document (communicate) the practitioners' evolving thought process and the patient's changing clinical course. Today's patient problem lists are cafeterias of unstandardized terms selected to meet the unwritten (!) requirement for a patient problem list. Psychiatric "patient problems" are typically adjectival descriptions (e.g., "attention-seeking behavior"), static conditions (e.g., "adoption issues"), critical judgments (e.g., "resistant to treatment"), theoretical constructs (e.g., "poor ego boundaries"), value statements (e.g., "poor peer choices"), anecdotal inferences (e.g., "demanding and dependent"), arbitrary conclusions (e.g., "poor impulse control"), or diagnoses (e.g., "dysthymia").

The problem list above, taken from an actual hospital record, fails to document (communicate) why the patient (admitted with the diagnosis of major depression) needed treatment at all, what treatment services were necessary, and why a particular intensity of service was required to carry out the services. A problem such as "adoption issues" contains no spectrum for change within its syntax, thereby paralyzing the practitioner's ability to communicate the patient's progress toward resolving the problem and to convey effectiveness of the treatment based on patient outcome.

Reviewers want to know how treatment decisions are made and what the clinical rationale is for each of them. An oft-heard comment from a reviewer is, "I may know what's going on with a patient, but I don't always know why." Again, this is because clinicians have not been educated about the value of articulating and documenting their own thought processes. The external review process inserts a number of questions between the time the practitioner establishes a diagnosis and the time he or she initiates the treatment. The reviewer wants to know why that treatment is necessary, why a particular level of care (intensity of service) is required, and why alternative treatments are not being considered. Lengthy problem lists and a multiplicity of treatment interventions do not provide this information.

We are committed to the belief that an easy-to-use, operational treatment language utilizing clear, commonly understood, behaviorally focused terms can communicate the measurable, objective process and quality of care to those individuals who need to know. Such a language does not require the mental health practitioner to forfeit or even necessarily compromise the appreciable, subjective quality of care—in all its subtlety and nuance—as currently understood and practiced. When practitioners can hear the questions asked by those who need to know as requests for clarity of thought, rather than as threats of nonpayment, they may well be able to artfully and more effectually respond to them as colleagues and not as menacing strangers.

Chapter 4

Patient Impairments and the Diagnosis

"What is the patient's diagnosis?"

Utilizing a common language of impairments to describe patients with mental disorders prepares the provider to communicate to the reviewer behavioral dysfunctions that can be readily understood. Impairments also become the reimburser's tools for making payment determinations. The advantages of impairments as behavioral descriptors of patient dysfunctions are discussed, and an open-ended dictionary of impairments that we have identified for patients receiving mental healthcare treatment services is presented.

The most commonly asked first question during an initial external review—for example, to obtain preauthorization for a hospitalization—is "What is the patient's diagnosis?" We agree with Kiesler (1982) that additional information is necessary to describe a patient's current psychiatric condition and explain the clinical rationale for the proposed treatment. The treatment language we have devised to link the patient's diagnosis to the mental healthcare practitioner's planned interventions is the subject of this chapter.

Diagnosis is the conclusive evidence of the treater's ability to synthesize findings. After obtaining a thorough history, performing mental status and physical examinations, and reviewing all available ancillary data (e.g., laboratory tests, consultation reports, narrative accounts by observers), the treater calls upon his or her skill, experience, and general fund of knowledge to formulate the nature of the condition—that is, the diagnosis. The practitioner then affixes the name of that condition to the patient. Establishing an accurate diagnosis informs the practitioner on how to proceed with treatment. More recently, diagnosis has also been employed to inform third-party payers and other external reviewers on how much to reimburse for certain treatment services.

The Medicare Prospective Payment System (PPS) fixes the reimbursement for hospital medical-surgical treatment to particular diagnosis-related groups (DRGs). The DRGs are based on the arguable premise that the descriptive label of a disorder—the diagnosis—is synonymous with or so closely approximates the afflicted individual and the treatment that will be given, that patient and diagnosis are interchangeable. Therefore, the costs to treat each are considered to be equivalent. Because the diagnostic nomenclature for describing psychiatric and chemical dependency patients does not by itself predict the treatment, psychiatry has maintained a DRG exemption from this mandated alliance between the diagnosis of a condition and the cost of treating a patient. As the DSM-III-R (American Psychiatric Association 1987) clearly cautions:

> A common misconception is that a classification of mental disorders classifies people, when actually what are being classified are disorders that people have . . .

> . . . Although all the people described as having the same
> mental disorder have at least the defining features of the
> disorder, they may well differ in other important respects
> that may affect clinical management and outcome. (p. xxiii)

Psychiatric diagnoses are descriptors of complex mental
states. Although certain diagnoses do in fact suggest specific
medication treatment protocols, the DSM-III-R nomenclature is
not by itself congruent with the type of service (e.g., individual
psychotherapy) or the intensity of service (e.g., hospitalization)
necessary to treat a patient in mental distress. In a study conducted 2 years after the publication of the DSM-III-R, it was found
that one-third of psychiatrists continued to use the DSM-III
(American Psychiatric Association 1980) as their primary diagnostic reference (Zimmerman 1988). A DSM-IV is now planned
for release by 1994 to maintain a consistent terminology and
coding system with the International Classification of Diseases—
10th Revision (ICD-10). Because patients can receive different
diagnoses depending on the system used, reviewers encounter
diagnoses that are now preceded by adjectives that are based on
a specific classification system (e.g., the patient has DSM-III
schizophrenia or DSM-III-R schizoaffective disorder).

At a practical level, clinicians are occasionally confronted
with the problem of explaining diagnostic changes to outside
reviewers. Reviewers get frustrated when they see multiple psychiatric diagnoses over time for the same patient. Trying to explain that a previous physician was using a different
nomenclature does not appease them. At the other end of the
spectrum, reviewers are also baffled when the entire patient
population on a psychiatric unit carries the diagnosis of "major
depression." These changing definitions of pathological conditions suggest the need for a consistent and descriptive language
of treatment that can be used to communicate to outside
reviewers the reasons (objectively manifest or subjectively
reported) why a patient needs care.

This is not an original idea. The psychiatric nursing profession has already conceptualized a compendium of treatment
descriptors for its own use. At the 1981 American Nursing Association Congress on Nursing Practice, the profession staked
its claim to diagnose and treat selected "health problems" using

behaviorally referenced "nursing diagnoses" that "objectify perceived difficulties or needs by naming them as bases for understanding and taking actions to resolve the concerns" (Kim et al. 1984, p. 26). These descriptors, endorsed by the North American Nursing Diagnosis Association (NANDA), represented the first organized effort to systematically catalog patient behaviors and link them to treatment intervention and outcome.

NANDA diagnoses structure the nursing care plan, and their concreteness and objectivity are valuable aids for monitoring and evaluating patient progress. In those psychiatric facilities where the written treatment plan is the responsibility of nursing professionals, these nursing diagnoses often become a generic treatment documentation language of their own. By definition and design, however, these terms are limited to the scope of the discipline. Some NANDA nursing diagnoses (e.g., "ineffective individual coping" and "alterations in thought process") are not serviceable to other mental health disciplines and either are precariously close to value judgments or represent inferential conclusions about static patient states or traits.

A number of exhaustive and comprehensive attempts have been made to systematize or codify a standard set of patient problems. However, the difficulty we found in a review of a number of dictionaries of psychiatric patient problems (e.g., Longabaugh et al. 1983; Meldman et al. 1976; POMR Project 1978) and several automated treatment planning programs for psychiatry (Angle et al. 1977; Ryback et al. 1981; L. McCullough and A. D. Farrell, unpublished manuscript, 1983) is that they all define "problem" with numerous parameters and overly broad guidelines. The resulting voluminous lists of terms only variably convince a reviewer why a patient needs particular services and why a specified level of service intensity is required to provide them.

Patient problem lists also do not systematically capture a patient's particular strengths and the comorbid conditions that may have an impact on the anticipated patient outcome for particular treatments. An articulate, motivated, responsible, and introspective patient may accomplish the outcome objectives and reach the goals of treatment in less time and at less expense than an individual who does not possess these particular strengths. On the other hand, an adolescent patient hospitalized for an acute schizophrenic episode who also has a learning disability, a major educational deficit, and lives with parents who are active substance abusers, may require more treatment efforts (at additional expense) than would be necessary to treat the schizophrenic episode without these additional comorbid conditions.

Based upon these observed shortcomings of current nosologies and organizational formats for documenting the treatment of psychiatric patients, we have developed a behavioral language for mental healthcare *treatment documentation* that has the following features:

1. Communicates the reason(s) for, and notarizes the appropriateness of, treatment.
2. Identifies the comorbid conditions and captures all adverse occurrences that may impact the course (and outcome) of treatment.
3. Is demonstrably behavioral, prompting practitioners to document (and communicate) objectified, behavioral progress toward patient outcome objectives.
4. Includes all the mental health issues identified in the DSM-III-R and psychiatric NANDA diagnoses.
5. Cogently, succinctly, and humanistically describes patient difficulties, from the initial visit (or preadmission screening) to the termination of treatment and follow-up.
6. Is serviceable to all practitioners, regardless of their theoretical or clinical orientation.
7. Coordinates a diversity of treatment modalities toward consensually agreed-upon patient dysfunctions and their remediation.
8. Can be easily learned and understood by individuals in all mental health disciplines and health professionals in other disciplines.
9. Is compatible with the biological, psychological, behavioral, and family and social system models that currently contribute to the understanding and treatment of psychiatric disorders.

We recommend that the behavioral dysfunctions for which patients appropriately seek and require mental health services primarily—and the identified conditions that may impact their treatment secondarily—be identified as patient "impair-ments." **Impairment** describes a worsening, lessening, weakening, damaging, or reduction in ability to function and, in turn, anticipates a potential for repair, improvement, enhancement, and strengthening. The impairments identified in this book were selected for their power to signal the appropriateness for treatment and frame the documentation and communication of not only the treatment plan but also the patient's response to treatment interventions.

Impairments can be regarded as the actional expressions of the DSM-III-R diagnoses, their psychodynamic explanations (e.g., "poor ego boundaries"), and their neurobiological origins (e.g., serotonin deficiency). **Impairments are the reasons why a patient requires treatment. They are not the reason(s) for the presence of the disorder, nor are they the disorder itself. Rather, they are observable, objectifiable manifestations that necessitate and justify care.** Impairments are "behavioral windows" into the aberrant biochemical phenomena and psychological variations of existence that are the etiology of psychiatric disorders. The treatment interventions prescribed for impairments are chosen for their ability to "repair" the disordered behaviors manifestly by correcting (ultimately) these biological dysregulations and experiential aberrations.

Comprehensive assessment of both the patient and the patient's operational world is necessary for restoration and maintenance of biopsychosocial completeness (Marmor 1982). This "holistic" approach is the basis for the "concentric sphere" paradigm we employ when describing the patient. Each "sphere" locates a number of potential impairments that mental healthcare practitioners may identify in patients whom they are assessing for treatment (see Figure 4-1).

Impairments may be located in both the patient's subjectively experienced "private" world and the objectively measured "public" or actional world. In our model, the patient's *biopsychology* is represented at the center, circumscribed by an anatomic skin boundary (which metaphorically encloses the patient's internal world or inner reality as well). Spheres "outside" of the patient (but still "within" his larger world)

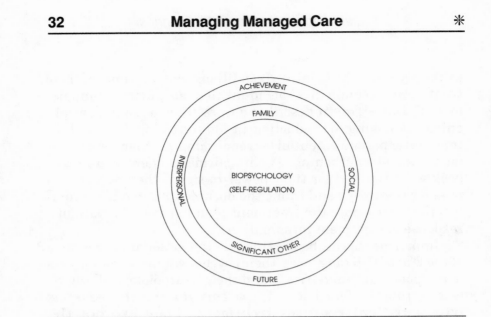

Figure 4–1. The internal and external world of the patient.

include the proximate and critically influential sphere of the *family/significant other* and the larger, developmentally postponed sphere of the *social/interpersonal*. Outermost is the sphere of *future/achievement*. The impairments that are assigned to each of these spheres are presented below. (See glossary in Appendix A for definitions of impairments.)

Biopsychology Impairments

The integrative concept of biopsychology updates a traditional demarcation between the body (biology) and the mind (psychology). The separation of "psyche" and "soma" is no longer metapsychologically explanatory or neurophysiologically valid. With respect to the psychoses, for example, it is now apparent that they may be either "psycho-somatic" or "somato-psychic" conditions (Grotstein et al. 1987). A psychosomatic alteration of the central nervous system following perceived catastrophic events may so alter the neurological mind that a secondary psychosomatic defect in mental processing is set in motion. The somatopsychic psychosis is an inherited defective neurological organization that is so fragile and hypersensitive to the stimuli of emotional experience that a disorganization of the central nervous system is too easily evoked. The consequence is a secondary psychic disorganization.

Biological givens (heredity) and experiential aberrations (environment) are conciliatorily understood in this model as reciprocal influences that are interdependent and interfacilitating. The impairments assigned to the sphere of biopsychology are no more than behavioral derivatives of (and windows to) neurophysiological, anatomical, biochemical, and experiential aberrations and their interplay. Hallucinations, for example, may be "explained" by the diagnosis of schizophrenia, which in itself is explained by neurobiological aberrations that lead to a faulty processing of experiential data, making "nonsense" out of "sense-ory" input from the real world (Flannery and Taylor 1981; Heilbrunn 1979; Meyersburg and Post 1979; Taylor 1985). To the outside reviewer, a diagnosis of schizophrenia implies a chronic, progressive disease. In our model, we do not include schizophrenia as an impairment because it does not communicate to a reviewer why a particular type of treatment is needed at a given point in time. That the patient is experiencing an impairment of hallucinations that, for example, are invoking thoughts of suicide is more to the point.

Impairments in the biopsychology sphere include behaviors that mediate between the patient's internal world and external reality in order to regulate, preserve, and restore psychological (and/or biological) homeostasis. These disordered behaviors are the actional (and at times desperate) efforts of the patient to maintain or restore psychological equilibrium in the face of painfully experienced tension states ranging from fleeting signal anxiety to profound dread, panic, and threats of psychological catastrophe. These tension states may spontaneously arise from within (neurophysiological dysregulation) or may be prompted by external stressors (environmental overload or deprivation). In either case, they impinge upon and threaten to harm the patient.

For example, obsessive-compulsive disorder was formerly understood only as a neurotic resolution of the anal phase of development and sadistic fantasies directed toward the object. Empirical psychobiological psychiatry now tells us that the "obsessive-compulsive neurosis" may also be a screen to defend against biological affective disorders, principally depressive or panic disorders (Behar et al. 1984; Elkins et al. 1980; Hoover and Insel 1984). The function of the obsessive-compulsive symptoms—and of phobias for that matter—is to circumscribe the area of biochemical defect and take active, fantasied measures (symptoms) to demarcate it and avoid it. Obsessive-compulsive disorder and other related disorders, therefore, may now be best treated with the combination of medication and psychotherapy. Such behaviors as bulimia and chemical dependence are also understood in this model as self-regulatory efforts "to feel good again" through the desperate behaviors of purging and liver cell destruction. When examined from this point of view, suicide is a desperate act contemplated or carried out to regulate oneself against such intolerable affect states.

The impairments we have defined as belonging to the sphere of biopsychology are listed in Table 4-1.

Table 4–1. Impairments in the biopsychology sphere

Altered sleep	Medical risk factor
Compulsions	Medical treatment noncompliance
Concomitant medical condition	Mood lability
Decreased concentration	Obsessions
Delusions	Paranoia
Deficient frustration tolerance	Pathological grief
Dissociative states	Pathological guilt
Dysphoric mood	Phobia
Dysphoric mood with alexithymia	Promiscuity
Gender dysphoria	Psychomotor agitation
Eating disorder	Psychomotor retardation
Encopresis	Psychotic thought and perception
Enuresis	Psychotic thought, perception,
Externalization and blame	and behavior
Fire setting	Rage reactions
Grandiosity	Self-mutilation
Hallucinations	Somatization
Hyperactivity	Stealing
Learning disability	Substance abuse
Manic thought/behavior	Suicidal thought/behavior

Family/Significant Other Impairments

Impairments in the patient's ability to relate to others are often the first ones to signal the patient's appropriate need for mental health services. While it is axiomatic that the role of the immediate family and significant other may be critical and even explanatory for the pathogenesis of patient dysfunctions, the presence of such difficulties may not by itself justify treatment at more intensive levels of care. Impairments in the family/significant other sphere are identified whenever such family interventions are able to facilitate whatever therapeutic progress is realistic or possible in a given clinical situation. Specific field resistances to patient progress may be reduced through selective family interventions (Brown 1980). Those interventions may occur occasionally, only once, or fairly often in the course of therapy with a designated patient. The progress toward meeting treatment goals for the biopsychology impairments may be aided through treatment of the patient's impairments in this sphere.

The impairments we have identified in the sphere of family/significant other are listed in Table 4-2.

Social/Interpersonal Impairments

Impairments in the social/interpersonal sphere document the patient's chaotic, confusing, unmanageable, or frankly overwhelming external world. This is a world characterized by destructive, dangerous relationships or behaviors that ulti-

---

Table 4–2. Impairments in the family/significant other sphere

Emotional/physical trauma perpetrator
Emotional/physical trauma victim
Family dysfunction
Family dysfunction with substance abuse
Marital/relationship dysfunction
Marital/relationship dysfunction with physical abuse
Running away

---

mately affect the patient and others. The treatment plan must respond to these difficulties in order to provide a consistent and durable environment in which the patient can improve overall functioning. It may be critical to the survival of the treatment (and the patient!) for the practitioner to intervene in destructive relationships and repair and facilitate healthy, supportive ones while treating the patient's biopsychology impairments. Impairments in the social/interpersonal sphere, such as oppositionalism or social withdrawal, will continue to compromise patient functioning in his or her world despite optimal treatment of, for example, the impairments of hyperactivity or psychotic thought and perception. The social/interpersonal impairments are often the comorbid conditions that ultimately determine the success or failure of treatment.

Impairments that we have identified in the social/interpersonal sphere are listed in Table 4-3.

Future/Achievement Impairments

In addition to the restoration of biopsychosocial completeness referenced above, there is a restoration of temporal completeness that we offer to our patients. We not only pay attention to what *was* (both constitutionally and experientially) and what *is* (behaviorally and biochemically), but we also address the treatable difficulties that obstruct or paralyze the patients' ability to plan and propel themselves into the future—for what *will be*. Impairments in the sphere of future/achievement, such as deficient frustration tolerance, hopelessness, and learning disability, impede and compromise the definition and achieve-

---

Table 4–3. Impairments in the social/interpersonal sphere

Assaultiveness	Paraphilia
Egocentricity	Repudiation of adults as helpers
Homicidal thought/behavior	Sexual dysfunction
Lying	Social withdrawal
Manipulativeness	Tantrums
Oppositionalism	Uncommunicativeness

Table 4–4. Impairments in the future/achievement sphere

Educational performance deficit	School phobia
Hopelessness	Truancy
Inadequate health care skills	Work dysphoria
Inadequate survival skills	

ment of personal goals and the actualization of potential. This is the sphere in which plans for the future, ambition for setting new goals, and the hope for tomorrow have either atrophied, become derailed, or been forfeited regardless of the cause. Impairments we have identified in the sphere of future are listed in Table 4-4.

It either has or will become obvious to the reader that the categorization of the impairments in the concentric sphere paradigm is somewhat arbitrary. The lists of impairments for each sphere are not intended to be definitively complete or exhaustive. These obvious shortcomings notwithstanding, we have found this model useful for the comprehensive identification of the problem areas in a patient's life that mental healthcare practitioners may address in their treatment plan. How we employ the impairment language to structure and organize the communication and documentation of all phases of patient care—from the initial intake assessment to the termination of treatment—is the subject of the remaining chapters in this book.

Chapter 5

The Patient Impairment Profile and Justification for Treatment

"Please tell me about the patient."

In this chapter the authors demonstrate the utility of the language of impairments for describing the reasons why a patient requires mental healthcare services. When taken together, all the identified behavioral dysfunctions (i.e., impairments) for which treatment will be provided comprise the Patient Impairment Profile. The authors present 12 clinical vignettes and detail the rationale for identifying the specific impairments for each patient.

The assessment of patients by systematically examining the "concentric spheres" of their internal and external worlds (see Chapter 4) encourages the identification of multiple impairments. In order to avoid the creation of a "stuffed problem list" that identifies every problem, potential or real, treatable or not treatable, we caution the practitioner to select only those impairments targeted for "repair" or treatment at a particular level of care. In our experience, a lengthy, or "stuffed," list of treatment concerns does a disservice to both the patient and the practitioner by blurring the specific reasons for which treatment is recommended. A large number of potential or, in some cases, unresolvable problems may not justify any treatment at all. And just one critically severe impairment *may* require, and be appropriately treated at, the most service-intensive level of care.

The major advantage of using the impairment language is having the capacity to describe in behavioral terms the patient's visible, quantifiable manifestations of the diagnosis. To this end, the selection of impairments is based upon the following criteria:

1. The impairment describes either patient behaviors or statements that can be objectified and quantified.
2. Only impairments that will be actively addressed in the treatment plan are selected.
3. The impairments selected are anticipated to improve with treatment.
4. The impairments are consistent with the DSM-III-R (American Psychiatric Association 1987) criteria for the patient's diagnosis.
5. All "spheres" of the patient's world are examined to identify any additional impairments that may have an impact on the treatment.

We recommend that the impairments be hierarchically listed, with the biopsychology impairments listed first. The impairment language is designed to communicate succinctly and accurately the clinical necessity for mental healthcare treatment services. A number of the impairments in these spheres *may* have levels of increased severity that provide further justification for a particular treatment or level of service (e.g., inpatient hospitalization). More will be said about rating the severity levels of the impairments in Chapter 6. The compilation of the impairments identified for treatment intervention becomes what we like to call the Patient Impairment Profile (PIP).

In our experience with external reviewers, the PIP provides a convenient outline to expeditiously respond to the often first-stated, and at times disquietingly vague, request, "Please tell me about the patient." Of course, the practitioner wants to know exactly what it is about the patient that the external reviewers would like to know. We have never found this type of request to be very helpful, because the guidelines that external reviewers use to determine clinical necessity are not always disclosed. Our response to this opening request is to state the patient's age, race, marital status, sex, and occupation and then proceed directly to the reasons why the patient is seeking treatment. We let the reviewer know that we have devised an impairment profile for the patient that identifies the acute clinical concerns that necessitate treatment. We indicate that we would like to refer to this list in the discussion of the patient throughout the course of treatment.

To those reviewers who choose to follow the traditional medical-surgical model by requesting the patient's diagnosis, we do provide the initial Axis I DSM-III-R diagnostic impression and then proceed as above. We do, however, avoid offering Axis II diagnoses (i.e., the personality disorders) for several reasons:

1. There is considerable confusion surrounding these diagnoses, which describe "persistent personality traits," and there is a lack of well-established validation of their diagnostic criteria and outcome with or without treatment (Vaillant and Perry 1985).
2. Some review organizations, without having clear research-based criteria on which to base their decision, do not include personality disorders as being eligible for mental health benefits.

3.   A growing body of literature is now reporting a temporal link between the major psychiatric disorders and the personality disorders (Othmer and Othmer 1989).

Offering the diagnosis of a personality disorder, unfortunately, suggests to some reviewers a chronic clinical condition and thus impedes the task at hand—which is to communicate (and document) why the patient needs treatment and why he or she needs it *now*.

The DSM-III-R V codes pose similar difficulties, and we avoid them as well. Their definition—"conditions not attributable to a mental disorder that are a focus of attention or treatment"—serves only to call into question why the patient requires *mental* healthcare services. Yet, the DSM-III-R is also quite clear in its discussion of the V codes that "with further information, the presence of a mental disorder may become apparent" (APA 1987, p. 359). And who is more skilled at making that determination than a mental health professional? As noted above, we have encountered some external review organizations that have identified personality disorders and V codes as either "red flags" for more indepth review or outright exclusion criteria for reimbursement. The offering of such "supplemental" diagnostic information can hamper the practitioner's communication of the clinical necessity for treatment.

Case Histories

Presented below are 12 clinical vignettes, selected to exemplify some of the more common patient difficulties that present to mental healthcare practitioners for treatment. The first five vignettes demonstrate the use of the PIP for patients requiring acute inpatient care. The second five illustrate the use of the PIP for patients receiving outpatient services. The last two vignettes show the utility of the PIP when used to describe chronic conditions with acute exacerbations that necessitate treatment.

The PIP that we developed for each of these clinical situations is provided, along with the Axis I and, where applicable, Axis II diagnoses, utilizing DSM-III-R criteria. The rationale for the selection of the particular impairments listed in each profile is presented. We wish to reiterate that the impairment language is not designed to compete or conflict with DSM-III-R nomenclature, which describes "disorders that people have" (APA 1987, p. xxiii). The impairment terminology is a behavioral treatment language for bridging the gap between diagnosis and the treatment interventions. Impairment language structures the communication and documentation about mental healthcare services and provides a clear rationale as to why those services are necessary.

We ask that special attention be given to the first two vignettes, Melanie W. and Bob D., because these two cases will be used as clinical examples throughout the remainder of the book to demonstrate the utility of the PIP for determining severity rating levels, creating patient outcome objectives ("goals" and "objectives"), and identifying treatment interventions (the treatment plan). The reader is again reminded that this language of impairments is neither definitive nor exhaustive; "impairments" other than those we have identified in Chapter 4 may be "created" by practitioners and should be included for their own use. What is essential is that any new term selected be demonstrably *behavioral* and contain *behavioral* manifestations with realistic potential for quantifiable improvement. The reasons for this will be expanded upon in subsequent chapters.

Case 1: Melanie W.

History

Melanie W., a 17-year-old high school student with juvenile-type diabetes mellitus, was referred for psychiatric hospitalization from a hospital facility specializing in chronic medical disease. Prior to her medical hospital admission, Melanie had been refusing to self-administer her insulin regularly, was frequently disregarding her diabetic diet, and, when angry or depressed, would "regulate" her mood by readjusting her insulin dose in order to precipitate severe hypo- or hyperglycemic episodes. She presented to the emergency room as a brittle, juvenile-onset–type diabetic whose blood glucose was measured at 415 mg/100 ml. Historically, Melanie's blood glucose was very difficult to control, and she had been hospitalized over 20 times for severe hyperglycemic episodes. When her condition was eventually stabilized in the hospital for her to adjust her twice-daily insulin doses on a fixed schedule based upon her blood glucose (which she tested herself in the morning and late afternoon), Melanie was referred for psychiatric evaluation after she stated that she could not make the commitment to responsibly follow this regimen on her own.

Melanie readily acknowledged her intent to deviate from the recommended insulin doses despite the potentially life-threatening consequences. She reported feeling "different from other kids" ever since she knew she had the disease and stated she did not care if she died early. She also admitted that she had no intention of curtailing intake of foods with high sugar content. Melanie was very knowledgeable about her diabetes, its management, and its clinical course, but she was unwilling to tailor her life-style to meet the demands of the illness.

Melanie's attendance at school had been erratic, and her educational performance had been very poor. The local school board was threatening legal action against the parents for tolerating, if not outrightly encouraging, Melanie's habitual truancy. Melanie's mother admitted that she was unable to get Melanie to go to school and, in fact, stated it was easier for her to have Melanie at home to help take care of Melanie's 8-month-old brother. Melanie saw no reason to attend school and had no future goals for herself, although she thought she might get married and have children someday.

Melanie's family life was very chaotic. She was the eldest of six children. Her father worked 6 days a week, 10 to 12 hours a day, and he unabashedly acknowledged that he was "not involved in the family" other than to complain about his wife's ineffectiveness with the children, the problems with which he felt his children burdened him, and the long hours of work necessary to support the family. Melanie's mother was quick to disclose that she was "quite disorganized" and was aware of her ineffectiveness in carrying out household responsibilities and in being a parent. Family chores were not defined, and the household ran on a crisis model. Although all eight family members lived in a three-bedroom home, Melanie had her own bedroom. The parents reported that this was due to Melanie's inability to get along with her siblings. Melanie, however, experienced this as further evidence that she was the "sick one" who needed to be isolated from the rest of the family. This isolation, in turn, reinforced her reclusiveness.

Clinical Presentation

Melanie presented as a moderately overweight high school student who was poorly groomed, unkempt, sullen, and slow to respond. Speech was visibly an effort for her, and she strained to find words, which she uttered just above a whisper. She was alert and coherent, although her use of language was somewhat childish.

She reported experiencing life as hopeless and seemed blandly indifferent to the life-threatening consequences of her intentional mismanagement of her diabetes. She looked puzzled when it was suggested that she might be angry about the severe imposition and limitations the diabetes exerted on her life. She said she never experienced anger and, in fact, stated that she didn't think she really knew what anger was. She denied any active suicidal intent, while at the same time acknowledging the seriousness and potential lethality of her behavior. There was no evidence of active psychosis or any organic impairment.

Assessment

Although Melanie denied active suicidal ideation, the impairment of suicidal thought/behavior was chosen because her behavior was indeed life-threatening, and Melanie would require close supervision to ensure her safety.

Melanie's depression manifested behaviorally with a visible and verbalized dysphoric mood, and her inability to label her range of affective experiences—alexithymia—would most probably encumber the treatment of the dysphoric mood. Her blatant refusal to manage her diabetes would require close medical supervision and psychotherapy. Her poor grooming, poor hygiene, and indifference to her diabetic management were three aspects of her inadequate healthcare skills that would require monitoring, education, and repair. The family dysfunction and truancy were self-evident. Melanie was admitted to an inpatient psychiatric unit with a diagnosis of major depression.

Patient: Melanie W.

Diagnosis:

Axis I: **Major depression, single episode, severe, without psychotic features (296.23)**

Axis II: **None**

Patient Impairment Profile:

1. Suicidal thought/behavior
2. Dysphoric mood with alexithymia
3. Concomitant medical condition (juvenile-type diabetes mellitus)
4. Inadequate health care skills
5. Family dysfunction
6. Truancy

[**Note to reader:** This is a frequently used diagnosis for psychiatric inpatients. When we reviewed the admissions to a 95-bed private psychiatric hospital over a 1-year period, we found that more than 75% of the patients were admitted and discharged with that diagnosis. Yet, the impairment profiles we had for these patients demonstrated a very diverse range of treatment concerns and approaches. The impairments are designed to be very patient-specific.]

Case 2: Bob D.

History

Bob was a 23-year-old male brought to a medical emergency room by his parents who were called by two of Bob's friends to tell them Bob had been "talking all night about performing, stating that he was a messenger from God." The friends reported that Bob was claiming that he could "move buildings and rearrange the city streets with his 'special' powers," and he was trying to convince them to break into a warehouse "so that he could convert it into a children's park." The parents picked Bob up and brought him to the emergency room for evaluation. They reported that Bob had been terminated recently from his job because of tardiness, absenteeism, and argumentativeness, and that he had been married for just over a year. Bob had previously lived at home after completing high school and one year of junior college. He had occasionally worked as an auto mechanic's assistant, but the parents confided that he had "never found a place to work where he was happy." Bob and his wife had continued to be largely dependent on his family for financial support. Bob's wife was also concerned about Bob's drinking "at least four to six beers a day" and his association with "people who didn't do much of anything but drink and 'hang out.'" Whenever attempts had been made by the family to discuss some of these behaviors with Bob, he became very angry, screamed obscenities, and would often storm out of the house and occasionally be gone for one or two days at a time. Any moderate impasse provoked such reactions.

Clinical Presentation

In the emergency room, Bob presented as a handsome, muscular, adult male, visibly agitated and obviously preoccupied. He could engage in the interview for only a minute or so before repeating very emphatically that he was God's chosen messenger and had been given the mission to save the children of the city by redesigning the streets and buildings. He smelled of alcohol, his speech was slurred, and he was moderately ataxic. He talked exuberantly about plans to perform "God's miracles" for "curing the sick and dying" and to "install more playgrounds and parks for children." He did not appear to be experiencing any hallucinations. There was no suicidal or homicidal ideation. He knew the month and the year, but not the date or day of the week. He became argumentative upon further questioning and stormed out of the room when psychiatric hospitalization was suggested. His parents were able to convince him, however, to sign himself in voluntarily.

Assessment

Although Bob presented with bizarre thoughts and behavior, the impairment of delusions was chosen over psychotic thought and behavior in order to describe more accurately the focal point of the initial treatment planned for him. The selection of the impairment of substance abuse (alcohol) is straightforward enough. Because of Bob's inability to manage the demands of full-time employment and the volatility and eruptive behavior he displayed when anyone tried to discuss particularly sensitive issues with him, and his similar behavior in the initial interview, the impairment of deficient frustration tolerance was included. While this is not an impairment that in itself necessitates hospitalization, the presence of Bob's deficient frustration tolerance would no doubt complicate his treatment. This comorbid condition would require its own specialized therapeutic interventions while Bob was in the acute treatment setting.

Patient: Bob D.

Diagnosis:

Axis I: **Psychotic disorder not otherwise specified (298.90); alcohol intoxication (303.00)**

Axis II: **None**

Psychiatric Impairment Profile:

1.   Delusions
2.   Substance abuse (alcohol)
3.   Deficient frustration tolerance

Case 3: Sarah C.

History

Sarah was a 13-year-old female admitted to the hospital because of her relentless carving on her arms and legs with kitchen tools and jackknives. Words, names of friends, and religious symbols were "tattooed" in scabs and scars on her forearms and lower thighs. She was also abusing alcohol daily and had been showing sudden changes in mood from vegetative social withdrawal to agitated, angry contrariness. These mood swings were increasing in frequency over the last half year. Sarah reported that she in fact enjoyed carving on herself, loved drinking alcohol, did not want to attend school, and hated her stepfather. The only thing she liked about "him and his rules" was the "fun in breaking them." She stated that she drank because it felt good and that she would stop "if my mother asked me to, but she never has." Sarah's mother presented as a very anxious, visibly overwhelmed woman who appeared frightened by her daughter. Sarah's mother herself had had a long history of depression, requiring numerous hospitalizations, and of being "too sensitive to medication to take any."

Sarah's biological father had died when Sarah was 11 years old; however, he and Sarah's mother had divorced when Sarah was 2. Sarah had continued to remain very close to her biological father, visiting him quite often until his death. Her mother had married Sarah's stepfather when Sarah was 6. Sarah now lived with her mother, maternal grandmother, and stepfather. He was a law enforcement officer and presented as gruff and authoritarian, with a narrow yet pragmatic view of the world. He and Sarah were obviously engaged in a power struggle, with her mother helplessly caught in the middle.

Clinical Presentation

Sarah presented as an unkempt, young Caucasian adolescent who looked several years older than her stated age. She was dressed in a "heavy metal" style—black chunky clothing, black ripped nylons, heavy jewelry—with one side of her head shaved. The baldness was covered by combing her very long hair across from the other side.

Sarah argued with any observation made about her, at times even contradicting her own statements made only minutes earlier. Simple requests (e.g., a physical exam, routine blood testing) were met with complaints, arguments, or frank refusal. She denied being actively suicidal, although she drank to the point of intoxication and carved on herself almost daily. No hallucinations, delusions, or organic impairments were evidenced.

At the end of the assessment, her mother also revealed that Sarah and her stepsister were dependents of the court because of parental neglect. The family had been investigated for the parents' failure to register the children in school, and the physical condition of the home was found to be unsafe and unsanitary.

Assessment

This is a severe and difficult case, with a number of acute problems identified in the profile justifying intensive, well-supervised treatment interventions. The criticalness of the self-mutilation and substance abuse is self-evident. A biological contribution to the mood lability would need to be considered, especially in light of the family history of affective disorder. Sarah's oppositionalism would need to be addressed as a specific treatment concern to facilitate repair of the more critical and severe impairments. The lack of family support and the absence of family structure (i.e., family dysfunction) made recidivism a major risk. The effects of the parental neglect on Sarah and her reactions to public investigation and being in legal custody of the court would also require exploration and understanding.

Patient: Sarah C.

Diagnosis:

Axis I: **Cyclothymia (301.13); rule out bipolar
             affective disorder (296.4x)**

Axis II: **Borderline personality disorder (301.83)**

Patient Impairment Profile:

1. Self-mutilation
2. Mood lability
3. Substance abuse
4. Oppositionalism
5. Family dysfunction
6. Emotional/physical trauma victim

[**Note to reader:** We believe this PIP accurately describes the concerns that the treatment team would be addressing while Sarah was in the hospital. Although the last three impairments are customarily treated in outpatient settings, in this case their presence impacted the treatment of the first three and hence are included in the profile.]

Case 4: George G.

History

George, a 19-year-old single high school graduate, was brought into treatment by his stepmother and father, who had become concerned about his increasing isolation from the family and few friends he had made while still in school. The parents also had noticed a deterioration in his personal hygiene over the last 6 to 8 months.

George had always verbalized his preference to remain at home and "help out the family." He never developed any outside interests and avoided any discussion with his family about emancipating himself or living on his own. George's parents had hoped he would "grow out of this" and were now concerned that he had not. George reported that he was frightened of people his own age, believing they would hurt him physically or make fun of him. He preferred the company of children 10 or more years his junior because "I can take care of them, and they like the same things I do."

He reported that life at home with his stepmother was without strife and that he was glad she and his father let him spend much of the day in his room daydreaming. George had disclosed to his stepmother that he had been physically abused by his biological mother and stepfather after his natural parents divorced when he was 3. When he was 8, George came to live with his biological father, who had remarried. George explained, "My real mother wanted me out of the house, and I wanted to live with my real father."

He reported that he felt safe in his new home but had never come to feel safe outside of it. School was always frightening for him. He had only a few acquaintances and never dated. After eight sessiohns of outpatient individual psychotherapy, George's condition was continuing to deteriorate.

Clinical Presentation

George presented as a timid, suspicious, tense, stiffly postured, less-than-tidy, thin, young adult male who was visibly uncomfortable in the interview. He spoke clearly but tersely and in a monotone. He reported feeling very lonely at times and remarked that he was even frightened by the interview. He denied any suicidal or homicidal ideation. He verbalized peculiar vague ideas regarding people and their motives—"People only talk to you if they want to get something out of you or hurt you."

In spite of his severe social withdrawal and very poor interpersonal skills, George verbalized some rather grandiose expectations for himself in life—"I don't have to work or go to school—my parents will always be there."

He denied experiencing any hallucinations, and there were no systematized delusions in evidence. He was oriented to time, place, and person. His immediate, recent, and remote memory were intact. He denied using alcohol or other drugs of abuse. His insights were very limited; his judgment was immature and poor.

Assessment

This case illustrates particularly well the effectiveness of the PIP for articulating a rationale for treatment. George's clinical presentation of a subchronic schizophrenic disorder does not by itself justify an "acute" diagnosis. The diagnosis, of course, describes only the category of disorders into which George's symptoms best fit. Yet, at the same time, he is clearly experiencing severe and compromising difficulties that warrant treatment intervention.

Whether the label for George's disorder is a schizophrenia (undifferentiated type or paranoid type) or a schizoaffective disorder is of less concern to an outside reviewer than the reasons why treatment is being recommended now. Not only did George fail to respond to outpatient treatment, but his impairments of paranoia, psychotic thought/perception, and social withdrawal were sufficiently disabling to warrant a more intensive level of care. The impairments of family dysfunction and emotional/physical abuse victim required treatment. By themselves, these impairments are usually treated in outpatient settings.

Patient: George G.

Diagnosis:

Axis I: **Schizophrenia, undifferentiated type, subchronic (295.91)**

Axis II: **Schizotypal personality disorder (301.22)**

Patient Impairment Profile:

1. Paranoia
2. Psychotic thought/perception
3. Social withdrawal
4. Inadequate health care skills
5. Family dysfunction
6. Emotional/physical trauma victim

Case 5: David C.

History

David, a 16-year-old male high school student, was brought in
for psychiatric evaluation by his mother, who had become
frightened by her son's violent behaviors. David and his mother
were interviewed conjointly first, then David was examined
individually. His mother reported feeling terrified by David's
volatile and explosive verbal assaults in response to what she
regarded as benign, noninvasive questions or requests (e.g.,
help with a household chore). While destruction of household
property (doors, furniture, glassware) was not uncommon,
there had been no physical altercations between David and his
mother. David reported feeling very guilty after each fight—
"after I had a couple of hours to cool down"—and although he
felt his mother was too intrusive and demanding, he stated he
knew that she was doing the best she could. David never knew
his father. David reported being frequently in fights in and
after school and openly admitted that he often hurt those he
fought. He typically believed it was "they" who started any
altercation (verbal or physical) and it was up to him to "finish
it—physically." On one occasion, he got into a fight with a gas
station attendant whom he had never met before. David knew
that he had seriously injured the man but had left before police
arrived. He only remembered being "flooded with anger" and

feeling completely out of control. David also reported difficulty keeping any part-time jobs because of his volatility. He often felt that "adults are always trying to take advantage of me." David verbalized feeling very depressed about himself, feeling that he was a "screw up and would probably only end up being a bum." He did not believe he could be a success at anything. He thought a great deal about dying, but denied any active suicidal ideation or plan. He had not been attending school and was thinking about dropping out altogether. Interestingly, David had joined a 12-step program and reported being free of drugs and alcohol for the last 8 months.

Clinical Presentation

David presented as a vigorous, handsome, muscular, stern-looking, and tensely postured adolescent who appeared "on the alert," suspicious, and ready to defend himself physically. His speech was fluent and coherent. His affect was broodingly serious, and he was easily angered. He never smiled. David was very self-deprecating and self-condemning, and he doubted that anyone or anything could be of help to him. He posited that dying was one way to escape the pain of living, but denied any specific plan. No overt psychotic thinking or organic impairment was in evidence.

Assessment

This complicated case is included to exemplify and clarify the differences in the use of the impairments of assaultiveness, rage reactions, and deficient frustration tolerance. Bob's behavior (case 2) was consistent with deficient frustration tolerance and was most accurately described by that term. Although David clearly did not tolerate much frustration either, the *behavioral* manifestations of that limitation—the rage reactions and the assaultiveness—more accurately describe David's difficulties and, hence, were chosen preferentially for inclusion in David's PIP. Additionally, the rage reactions that characterized the difficult interactions with his mother were quite different (and would require different treatment interventions and different outcome objectives) from the assaultiveness behavior that David reported in the interview.

Patient: David C.

Diagnosis:

Axis I: **Major depression, single episode, with psychotic features (296.24); intermittent explosive disorder (312.34)**

Axis II: **None**

Patient Impairment Profile:

1.   Paranoia
2.   Rage reactions
3.   Assaultiveness
4.   Dysphoric mood
5.   Inadequate survival skills
6.   Family dysfunction

[**Note to reader:** It is important to note, also, that we do not include the familiar term "poor impulse control" as an impairment to describe these kinds of behaviors. Poor impulse control is a theoretical explanation of objectionable behavior based upon "drive model" psychoanalytic metapsychology, and we find the term overused and often misunderstood. The question to be asked when confronted with such an "explanation" is "What happens when there is a loss of 'impulse control'?" The answer to that question is the basis for selecting the appropriate impairment.]

Case 6: Jerry D.

History

Jerry was a 28-year-old male electrician who sought treatment for alcohol abuse and a failing marriage. He reported drinking daily since his early teens and currently drank at lunch hour, on work breaks, and most nearly every evening. He only attended social engagements where alcohol was served and, more often than not, would become intoxicated. At least once a week he experienced a blackout, not remembering when or even how he got home. Jerry nervously revealed that his wife had recently moved out of the house and was threatening divorce.

Since then he reported feeling very lonely, helpless about how to restore his relationship with his wife, and full of worry as to how he would ever find another "girl of my dreams." He wanted his wife to become involved in treatment with him to work on their marital problems. Jerry had tried attending Alcoholics Anonymous and even obtained a sponsor to help him develop a program of sobriety, but he was unable to stay sober. He was frightened about hospitalization, but thought he needed it and didn't know what else to do. His wife agreed to participate in his rehabilitation treatment program.

Clinical Presentation

Jerry presented as an attentive, polite, nicely groomed male who was motivated to save his marriage and distressed about his alcohol abuse and the effect it was having on his relationship with his wife. Although at times he felt helpless and hopeless in the face of his problems, he denied any suicidal ideation or plan. He indicated that some of his friends noticed he was withdrawing from them and that he often appeared to be sad and preoccupied. There was no evidence of a thought disorder or organic impairment.

Assessment

Although Jerry was feeling hopeless about his marital situation and it was in turn affecting his ability to work on his alcohol abuse problem, he did not meet the criteria for a DSM-III-R mood disorder. And, yet, he did exhibit a number of observable behaviors consistent with a dysphoric mood. The substance abuse was clearly out of Jerry's control and endangering his life (the blackouts). Jerry's dysphoric mood was manifested by his inability to concentrate (daydreaming), worry, and feelings of sadness and futility. Even though Jerry was admitted to an inpatient alcohol rehabilitation program, the dysphoric mood and marital dysfunction would impact the clinical course of his alcohol abuse rehabilitation and would therefore require additional, specific treatment interventions as well.

Patient: Jerry D.

Diagnosis:

Axis I: **Alcohol abuse (305.00)**
Axis II: **None**

Patient Impairment Profile:
1. Substance abuse (alcohol)
2. Dysphoric mood
3. Marital relationship dysfunction

Case 7: Darryl C.

History

Darryl, an 8-year-old boy, was referred for psychiatric evaluation by his third-grade teacher because he was "acting odd and depressed" in the classroom. Darryl's mother accompanied him to the interview. She reported that Darryl had always been a loner, a child who preferred to be at home with her rather than with children his age. Whenever mother had tried to encourage him to interact with anyone outside his family, Darryl would either burst into tears, saying he was afraid, or else immediately refuse and retreat to his room. His mother indicated that he appeared most happy when engaged at his computer, where he could entertain himself for hours on end and into the night with computer games, computer drawing, and science education tutorials.

Darryl had been identified as a very bright, intellectually gifted child with special interests and talent in mathematics and science. In the last year, Darryl became preoccupied with the idea that because he could learn math and science on a computer, there was no reason for him to go to school at all. He persevered in repetitive, incessant debates with his parents to convince them of this fact. His mother and father both sensed that Darryl was becoming increasingly fearful of outsiders. At times they had found him in his room crying, and on one occasion Darryl asked his mother what she thought about people who kill themselves. Darryl had one sister, 3 years younger, who appeared to be developing normally.

Clinical Presentation

Darryl presented as an unanimated, almost mannequin-like, 8-year-old, who sat rigidly erect in his chair, not moving a muscle, staring directly into the interviewer's eyes. He was garrulous and very proficient in his use of language, but his speech was stilted. Darryl's "conversation" sounded more like a practice recitation in front of a mirror—how one might sound when talking to one's self.

Darryl acknowledged he often felt sad and occasionally cried, but stated that he did not know the reason why. He could always make himself feel better by sitting down at his computer. He had frequent thoughts about dying but stated that he did not want to hurt his mother.

He regarded himself as intellectually superior to his peers and reported he had no interest in any of the things children his age liked to do. He felt "picked on" by his classmates but at the same time was insensitive to the provocativeness of his repeated critical attacks on them as being "intellectually inferior." Darryl was quick to add that if he were asked by anyone to do something he did not want to do (e.g., read aloud in class or play some particular game with a peer), he would become "very upset" and be desperate in his room at his computer. He stated that he never had any use for fairy tales and found them boring.

Although Darryl was impressively knowledgeable about computer and other sciences, he was conspicuously uninformed about social norms and conventions of social interaction. The logic of his attending school rather than learning about life through a computer eluded him.

Assessment

Darryl's diagnostic formulation was tentative, and the case could be made that Darryl was actually demonstrating a schizophrenic disorder rather than psychotic depression and autistic behaviors. We point out here that the PIP accurately captures the behavioral dysfunctions that will be addressed in treatment regardless of the patient's "final" diagnosis.

Patient: Darryl C.

Diagnosis:

Axis I: **Major depression, single episode, with
psychotic features (296.24)**

Axis II: **Autistic disorder (299.00)**

Patient Impairment Profile:

1. Psychotic thought and perceptions
2. Dysphoric mood
3. Inadequate survival skills
4. Social withdrawal

Case 8: Jason K.

History

Jason was an 11-year-old boy brought in for evaluation by his
parents after he threatened to kill himself with a knife. For the
last several months, Jason had been refusing to go to school
and when coerced to do so would have such tantrums that it
was impossible to get him out of the house. In the last several
weeks, Jason would conclude his tantrums with a threat to kill
himself. On the evening prior to the evaluation, his parents had
discovered that Jason had a knife with him in his bed. Jason
threatened that he might use it if they tried to take it away.
Jason had been voicing his resistance to going to school for
2 years. He never gave any reasons for this; yet, more and
more frequently, when he did go to school he would be in the
school nurse's office by midmorning, in tears, complaining of a
headache or a stomachache, wanting to go home. The parents
felt helpless.

They reported that Jason enjoyed playing baseball with his
friends, as long as he was close to his home, and that he enjoyed
family activities as well. On one occasion, Jason did say that
he was worried some harm might befall his mother when he
was not at home. Whenever Jason was asked to do something
he did not want to do, he would yell, stamp his feet, strike out,
throw things against the walls, kick the walls, slam doors,
curse, and, most recently, threaten to kill himself.

Clinical Presentation

Jason presented as a small-for-his-age, 11-year-old who clearly gave the impression of being at the evaluation under duress. His answers to questions were skimpy, at times curt. Whenever he had the opportunity to disagree, he would become vigorously vocal and animated. Several times he disagreed with his own previous statements, yet this never daunted him. He would only state that he hated school and just wanted to stay home and play. Jason denied periods of sadness or loneliness, and he denied having made statements regarding suicide or of having the knife in his bed. These "disclaimers" seemed more contrary than dishonest or amnestic. There were no psychotic processes in evidence. His intellectual functioning was unimpaired.

Assessment

Even though school refusal in DSM-III-R is understood as being symptomatic of a separation anxiety disorder rather than a discrete disorder, we chose to include school phobia as an impairment because it is an effective descriptor of Jason's behavior (Appendix A) and is quantifiable and contains a spectrum for change that can be behaviorally measured. We chose to include both the tantrums and the oppositionalism because, while the tantrums are the end result of an oppositional encounter with an adult, Jason's arguing and defiant refusal of adult requests would require different treatment interventions (see Chapter 9) apart from and after the resolution of the tantrums.

Patient: Jason K.

Diagnosis:

Axis I: **Separation anxiety disorder (309.21);**
         oppositional defiant disorder, severe (313.81)

Axis II: **None**

Patient Impairment Profile:

1. Suicidality
2. School phobia
3. Tantrums
4. Oppositionalism
5. Family dysfunction

[**Note to reader:** Is Jason depressed? This is an interesting question that highlights the multiplicity of meanings of the term that are often not clarified in discussion. Aren't most, if not all, actively suicidal patients depressed? That Jason is a suicide risk is clear from his behavioral presentation, and, hence, we included it in the PIP as an impairment. While there is a manipulative quality to his threats of suicide, they are nonetheless still desperate statements and conjure associations of helplessness and hopelessness. And yet, Jason does not demonstrate any visible signs or symptoms of a dysphoric *mood*—for example, psychomotor retardation, any statements of hopelessness, or any expressions of sadness, feeling blue, or feeling lonely. Jason was not phenomenologically depressed. At the same time, we are inclined to believe that Jason's phobia, tantrums, and oppositionalism were all attempts at mastering a "depressive core" that is the basis of a separation anxiety disorder. If, after successful treatment of the phobia, tantrums, and the oppositionalism impairments, the "depression" is unmasked and reveals itself behaviorally, *then* the impairment of dysphoric mood may be added to the profile (with the successfully "repaired" impairments having been deleted from it).]

Case 9: Nancy D.

Clinical Presentation

Nancy was a 30-year-old single female who presented at her internist's office with complaints of severe chest constriction. Upon examination, she was told that she had a "mild pneumonia" that could be easily treated on an outpatient basis. Nancy became irate and stormed around the room, yelling that she felt like she was going to die, terrified that her lungs might "fill up again," and that she needed to be in the hospital. She demanded to use the telephone to find another doctor who would hospitalize her. When the internist tried to reassure and calm her, she became even more agitated and left the examining room. She then began badgering the receptionist to "please get me into a hospital," screaming that no one understood how badly she felt, that she could not sit still a minute longer, and that she "had not slept in 2 days." "My legs won't stop dancing!"

she pleaded. Nancy was unable to process any sentences longer than four or five words because she became so agitated and distraught. She became threatening and accusing when confronted about the inappropriateness of her behavior by the receptionist, and she refused to leave the office unless she got her way. The internist then consulted a psychiatrist, and together they admitted her to a psychiatric facility. The patient's health insurance plan required preauthorization for hospitalization except in the case of medical emergency.

Assessment

This case is included to illustrate the PIP as a vital, dynamic document that, when examined retrospectively, recounts the evolving evaluation and treatment process in "difficult to diagnose" cases. Nancy's severe psychomotor agitation and its profound interference with even the most rudimentary basic functioning argued for prompt, intensive intervention. Admitting a patient to "rule out" a diagnosis of a bipolar disorder does not communicate adequately why the patient needs treatment.

Patient: Nancy D.

Diagnosis:

Axis I: **Rule out bipolar disorder, manic, severe,
              with psychotic features (296.33)**

Axis II: **None**

Patient Impairment Profile:

1.   Psychomotor agitation

After Nancy was hospitalized, more information was obtained. Nancy had in fact been recently discharged from another medical facility for treatment of a pulmonary fat embolism following an outpatient surgical procedure she had had earlier that same day—hence, the fear of her lungs "filling up" again. While on the psychiatric unit, neurological evaluation subsequently concluded that Nancy had also probably suffered a basal ganglia infarct following the embolism, resulting in the parkinsonism that was responsible for her shuffling, agitated gait—her "dancing legs." It was also discovered that about a year prior to her psychiatric admission, she had been treated as an outpatient for a manic episode but had discontinued her medication and therapy about 4 months ago. Once the explanation for her psychomotor agitation impairment was found, Nancy's PIP was revised:

Patient Impairment Profile (update):
1. Psychomotor agitation (revised) (see 2, 3, and 4 below)
2. Manic behavior
3. Concomitant medical condition (parkinsonism, secondary to basal ganglia infarct, posttraumatic)
4. Medication noncompliance

Case 10: Richard J.

Clinical Presentation

Richard, a 29-year-old married male construction worker, sought treatment to repair a failing marriage. He indicated that his wife had threatened to leave him, and, when faced with this possibility, he found himself becoming increasingly irritable. Richard also began to dread what life would be like without her and felt anxious that life might "never be the same." He was angry that his wife was spending more and more time away from home and accusatorily complained that she was now consuming alcohol almost daily. He acknowledged that he also drank daily, "but not as much as she did."

His wife Carolyn reported a long history of struggling with her husband to improve their communications. She stated that from the beginning of their 6-year marriage, he would frequently work late into the evening, often failing to keep his promise to call her when he knew this was going to occur. She stated that they quickly lost the common friends and interests they shared prior to getting married. As a result, she began spending more and more time with single friends from work and, in the last few months, had on occasion drunk until she either passed out or blacked out. Two weeks ago, she decided to take the advice of friends and attended several Alcoholics

Anonymous meetings. At the time of the interview, she had 1 week of sobriety. She felt that in order to be successful with her sobriety plan, it was important for her husband never to drink in her presence. She also wondered whether the marriage was salvageable because she was not sure if she cared anymore. The years of trying to make her husband pay attention to her and the years of trying to have a social life without her husband had left her distant from him, and she did not want to be hurt and unhappy anymore.

Assessment

Richard actually sought treatment because of despondent concerns about his failing marriage that were causing him a great deal of anxiety. His diagnoses do not completely and accurately communicate the nature of his difficulties—which an outside reviewer would need to know before authorizing marital therapy for him. Whether he has a primary alcohol abuse problem was at the time of the initial evaluation unclear; however, his drinking was clearly compounding the marital difficulties and, as a result, increasing his agitation and worry about the future, hence its inclusion in the PIP.

Patient: Richard J.

Diagnosis:

Axis I: **Atypical depression (311.00);
alcohol abuse (305.00)**

Axis II: **None**

Patient Impairment Profile:

1. Psychomotor agitation
2. Substance abuse (alcohol)
3. Marital dysfunction

Case 11: Beatrice D.

History

Beatrice was a 73-year-old woman referred for evaluation by the owners of the board and care facility where she resided because "she's talking to imaginary people, physically attacking her roommate without apparent provocation, and refusing to eat or take her high blood pressure pills." She had resided there for 7 years, had never been a management problem, and took no other medications. Also, Beatrice's personal hygiene had become increasingly poor over the last several months. No other information was available at the time of evaluation.

Clinical Presentation

Beatrice presented as an elderly, unkempt, disheveled, adequately nourished, well-hydrated, elderly female who was visibly suspiciously and furtively looking about the room. Her speech was fluent, and she shouted repeatedly that she was being "taken away from my home." She blamed her caregivers for all her current difficulties. She was excitable and at times refused to talk. Beatrice refused to answer any questions regarding her mood, folding her arms across her chest and staring away from the interviewer. She did state, however, that several "little people" had been coming into her room now and then and occasionally moved and rearranged her furniture and belongings around. She didn't mind that, however, and said she enjoyed talking to her "little friends." She acknowledged becoming irate whenever anyone else came into her room—"They were stepping on my little friends!"—and she felt the need to protect her "little friends" by pummeling her intruders. She also reported hearing voices but did not know where they came from. They were male voices and usually just called her name. Beatrice did not know the date, the day of the week, or the month. She became angry when asked her address or the name of the facility where she was residing. Beatrice knew her birthday. When asked to remember the names of two unrelated objects, after a few minutes of distraction, she could not recall them.She could recall three numbers forward and two numbers backward. Blood pressure was 180/100 and pulse was 80 and irregular, and she was afebrile.

Assessment

Beatrice was obviously psychotic, a danger to others, and unable to care for herself. The reasons for this in the absence of any psychiatric history were unclear. Her elevated blood pressure was probably the result of her lack of compliance with her medical regimen. Beatrice was admitted to the hospital for medical, neurological, and psychiatric evaluation.

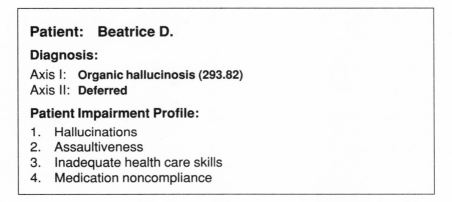

Patient: Beatrice D.

Diagnosis:

Axis I: **Organic hallucinosis (293.82)**
Axis II: **Deferred**

Patient Impairment Profile:
1.   Hallucinations
2.   Assaultiveness
3.   Inadequate health care skills
4.   Medication noncompliance

[**Note to reader:** This case is included to illustrate a not unfamiliar clinical presentation that is often subject to more rigorous external review. Subsequent neurological evaluation concluded that Beatrice was suffering from Alzheimer's disease (ICD-9 331.0) (which would be coded on Axis III). The diagnosis "organic hallucinosis" suggests to reviewers the presence of an "organic brain syndrome," which, in turn, suggests chronicity. A chronic condition does not by itself justify acute care. We used the PIP listed above to structure the communication of the acuity of Beatrice's difficulties. In this particular case, we prefer to use the impairments of hallucinations and assaultiveness rather than psychotic thought/perception and behavior because the former are more specific, accurate descriptors of the difficulties that necessitated treatment.]

Case 12: Peter K.

History

Peter, a 45-year-old male bus driver, had recently moved from another state to his present residence. After the move, he sought out a new psychiatrist, who gave him chlorpromazine, which he had been taking since his last psychiatric hospitalization 2 years earlier. Peter had had seven hospitalizations for acute schizophrenic episodes since the age of 19. In the acute phases of his illness, he would become extremely paranoid, delusionally jealous, severely agitated, and on three occasions physically threatening. For the last 2 years, he has maintained himself on chlorpromazine, 200 mg a day, without relapse. He has been able to work full-time as a bus driver for the city's transportation department and takes good care of his personal and financial responsibilities. He has lived alone since moving out of his parents' home when he was 24. Peter was able to identify the specific social situations that made him feel paranoid and/or fearful of losing control, and he avoided them as much as possible. He acknowledged he occasionally had difficulty determining how much of his feeling persecuted was real, and wished to know how much additional chlorpromazine he might need to take and for how long.

Assessment

Although Peter's condition is in remission at this time, he still considers psychotherapy treatment to be necessary to help him continue to sort out what is real and not real, both in his thoughts and in his perceptions. He also notes that the medication is particularly helpful when he begins to feel paranoid, and he titrates this symptom with an additional 50 to 150 mg of chlorpromazine a day. The PIP guides the outside reviewer to the issues that require both ongoing psychotherapy and medication maintenance management.

Patient: Peter K.

Diagnosis:

Axis I: **Schizophrenia, paranoid type, unspecified, stable (295.30)**

Axis II: **None**

Patient Impairment Profile:

1.   Psychotic thought, perception, and behavior
2.   Paranoia

After the justification for treatment is established, the practitioner needs to provide convincing information to support the type and intensity of treatment being recommended for the patient. The usefulness of the PIP for structuring this discussion with reviewers and documenting "How sick is the patient?" is the subject of Chapter 6.

Chapter 6

Impairment Severity
and Appropriateness
of Treatment

"Can the patient be treated at
a lower level of care?"

The assignment of a severity of illness rating for acute medical-surgical care diagnoses is now legislatively mandated in 19 states. Severity ratings can also be determined for each impairment, based upon specific patient behaviors. The authors define four levels of severity that are used to rate selected critical impairments; the less serious impairments are rated by either of the two lower levels of severity.

The clinical vignettes presented in Chapter 5 illustrate the utility of the Patient Impairment Profile (PIP) for accurately communicating and documenting the nature of a patient's dysfunctions, while also justifying the need for mental healthcare treatment services. Once the clinical necessity for treatment is established, the next question to be addressed is "What level or intensity of care is most appropriate for treating the patient?" Mental healthcare practitioners must effectively communicate just how impaired a patient is in order to justify a particular level of care. The severity of the identified impairment(s) determines the need for, and answers questions concerning the appropriateness of, more intensive levels of care (e.g., hospitalization).

"Severity of illness" is the degree of risk of immediate death or permanent loss of function due to a disease (or impairment). The severity of the illness is closely linked to what is often referred to as the "intensity of service"—that is, the level of care necessary to most appropriately and effectively treat the patient. The reasoning behind this is that the more severe an acute illness is, the more intense will be the level of service necessary to return the patient to wellness. The term "case complexity" is also now being employed to address severity of illness, although these two concepts are not quite the same. Patients who are "complex" (i.e., have multiple impairments or a complicated impairment profile) may or may not be severely ill in the previously defined sense of immediate risk of death or permanent loss of function. Therefore, we shall continue to use severity of illness (for our purposes, the severity of the impairment) as it relates to more costly, acute care for a particular illness.

The current diagnosis-related group (DRG) Medicare Prospective Payment System (PPS) does not adequately take severity of illness into account. As a result, hospitals that treat a greater proportion of more severely ill patients may sometimes "appear" to have higher costs, lower productivity, and poorer quality of care, when actually the explanation lies in the fact that their patient population may be genuinely sicker. Severely ill patients are often critically ill and require more costly care in intensive care units. A real concern is that some hospitals might have to refuse to treat these sicker patients if DRG payments do not cover treatment costs. One proposed solution to this dilemma is to adjust the DRGs with an appropriate severity of illness measure so that critically ill patients are appropriately classified, cared for, and paid for. The Yale School of Management, under a Health Care Financing Administration (HCFA) contract, has developed a system called the DRG Refinement algorithm to do this. The DRG Refinement collapses the currently used 475 DRGs into approximately 385 "refined groups," each of which has either three or four severity levels. It is believed that the HCFA will seek congressional approval to adopt the DRG Refinement as part of the Medicare prospective payment for fiscal year 1992.

While mental healthcare services continue to operate under a DRG exemption, we have found that in communicating the seriousness of a patient's impairment(s) to external reviewers, the level of severity of the impairment(s) is the decisive factor in obtaining preauthorization or concurrent authorization for more intense (and usually more costly) levels of service (e.g., hospitalization, a 5-day-a-week day treatment program, or individual psychotherapy more frequently than once a week).

There is another line in the historical development of the current concepts of severity of illness with which mental healthcare practitioners should be familiar. After the implementation of the Medicare PPS, it became possible for hospitals to combine clinical patient information and financial information (charge data) for studying the appropriateness of hospital use (utilization), for improving charge comparisons across hospitals and departments within hospitals, and for strategically planning budgets. Several major accounting firms developed automated "case mix" management systems to help hospitals do this. Medicare patients' DRGs were matched with charge data to compare practitioner utilization of resources and ordering practices. The objection was immediately raised, of course, that some practitioners' patients were receiving more resources because they were "sicker"—that is, more severely ill. Unless these more severely ill patients were identified and the degree of their severity factored into the monitoring data, accurate determinations of appropriate practitioner utilization would continue to require in-depth, time-consuming, and costly manual review of each case and each practitioner.

To fill the need for severity-adjusted utilization monitoring and to facilitate compliance with the requirement of the Joint Commission that hospitals and medical staffs carry out quality monitoring and peer review, over a half-dozen companies have developed computerized severity-of-illness systems that can be used to evaluate clinical data and then assign each case an arbitrary severity "score" or "rating." In several of the more widely used systems, the scores range from "0" (i.e., no significant clinical findings or complications) to "4" (i.e., critical findings indicating the presence of organ failure or death). In some systems, an additional severity level of "5" is used to signify death. At this time, there is no "gold standard" against which each of these severity systems can be functionally measured and evaluated. Severity of illness is defined somewhat differently in each of these systems. Each system uses its own scales, which are not comparable across systems. Each system also has different fixed and variable costs.

This bewildering lack of uniformity of standards with respect to how sick a patient needs to be in order to be treated appropriately and effectively at a more intensive level of service is conspicuously evident in the utilization guidelines that external review organizations use as well. There appear to be as many criteria and guidelines determining appropriate intensity of treatment for mental disorders as there are utilization review organizations. The challenge for the mental healthcare practitioner is to be able to communicate and document as accurately as possible the seriousness of their patients' difficulties in order to justify the particular level of care for which they are seeking approval.

Notwithstanding the absence of the "last word" in severity-of-illness determination, 19 state legislatures have already proceeded to mandate that their hospitals' published charge data be adjusted for severity of illness (using a particular severity-of-illness system that each state chose on its own) in order to obtain comparative cost and quality information for all the hospitals and practitioners located in their state. Again, in part as a result of the DRG exemption for psychiatry, the focus of these mandates is currently on acute medical and surgical care. Three of the severity-of-illness systems we reviewed, however, do contain severity ratings for the nervous and mental diseases found in the *International Classification of Diseases, 9th Revision—Clinical Modification* (ICD-9-CM). The severity-of-illness concept is as relevant to mental healthcare treatment services as it is to acute medical-surgical care. We have responded to this by applying the severity-of-illness concept to the PIP.

The same concerns we detailed in Chapter 3 regarding the utility of the DSM-III-R diagnoses for communicating the nature of the patient's difficulties also apply when trying to articulate the severity of the patient's illness. It made sense to us that the impairments could also be rated by their severity at the initiation of treatment and be reassessed at periodic intervals thereafter. We decided to identify four levels of severity in order to be consistent with the most widely used severity-of-illness systems currently employed throughout the country. These levels of severity are defined as follows:

> **Level 4: Imminently dangerous**
> **Level 3: Incapacitating**
> **Level 2: Debilitating**
> **Level 1: Moderate**
> **Level 0: Absent, nonpathological**

In order to maintain the focus of the impairment language on the patient and the patient's aberrant behaviors, we have defined quantifiable patient behaviors and/or patient statements for each of these levels of severity. We must emphasize that these levels of severity do not necessarily coincide with, indicate the need for, or even imply a particular intensity of service. An impairment of Level 4 severity may or may not require an intensive inpatient care setting. Outpatient crisis management models may be equally effective and appropriate. It is important to reiterate that the behavioral definers of these severities are the patient's and not the treater's. Statements such as "The patient requires one-to-one supervision" do not accurately convey enough convincing patient behavioral information to external reviewers to ensure approval for intensive treatment services. "The patient needs acute stabilization on antidepressants" is a treatment intervention required because of the severity of the patient's impairment(s). As repeated throughout this book, external reviewers need to know *why* the proposed treatment is necessary, in addition to knowing what the specific treatment is going to be for each patient.

Global generic patient behaviors for each severity level are presented below. The presence of either one or more than one of these behaviors justifies that severity rating for the particular impairment. In most cases, these definers will require elaboration and "translation" into specific patient behaviors when the severity level of a particular impairment is being determined. In the two case examples included at the end of this chapter, we present patient behavioral parameters that corroborate each level of severity for the patient's impairments. We apply these parameters to the patient clinical data and then determine the severity levels for those impairments.

Severity Levels

An impairment rated at **Level 4** (imminently dangerous) defines an impairment that is *imminently* destructive or life threatening to the patient and/or others. Such behaviors can be broadly defined to include:

* Active suicide threats or behavior
* Active violent or destructive behavior
* Active endangering runaway behavior or risk
* Demonstrable absence of, or severely compromised, reality testing
* Total inability to perform self-care skills
* Disruptive or isolative behavior that prevents participation in treatment

An impairment rated at **Level 3** (incapacitating) defines an impairment that renders the patient *acutely* incapable of normal activity (disabled) and/or potentially dangerous to self and/or others. Such behaviors can be broadly defined to include:

* Recent suicide behavior, threat, or current ideation
* Recent violent-destructive behavior or current ideation
* Recent endangering runaway behavior or current ideation

✴ Severely compromised healthcare skills
✴ Frequent bizarre thoughts or behavior
✴ Frequent disruptive or isolative behaviors that impede treatment

An impairment rated at **Level 2** (debilitating) defines an impairment that *markedly compromises* independent, vocational, and community functioning and/or inhibits the effectiveness of family-social support systems in "repairing" the impairment.

An impairment rated at **Level 1** (moderate) defines an impairment that is present and has the potential for repair or an impairment that, though presently absent, has a predictable likelihood of occurrence or recurrence without treatment. Again, the impairment terminology by definition communicates the justification for treatment at some level of care.

An impairment rated at **Level 0** (absent, nonpathological) is an impairment that has either been completely repaired or abated to such a low level that treatment intervention is no longer required.

Critical Impairments

Not all of the impairments listed in Chapter 4 have levels of severity that are incapacitating or imminently dangerous within the behavioral context of their definitions. Some impairments may "appear" to be more severe, when, in fact, this apparent severity is more correctly explained by the presence or emergence of another impairment. Some examples should clarify this point. If a patient with an identified impairment of inadequate healthcare skills subsequently develops delusions that place the patient in critical danger (an elderly diabetic patient, for example, develops the delusion that he is immortal and hence cured of the diabetes, no longer requiring insulin), it is the severity of the delusions that places the patient in imminent danger (in this case, Level 4 severity). Rating the delusions, rather than the inadequate healthcare skills, as a 4 is more consistent with, and more accurately communicates, the acute treatment concerns.

If the impairment of deficient frustration tolerance becomes manifested and expressed by verbalized threats to physically harm others, it is the impairment of assaultiveness that is identified as potentially dangerous. For example, when an adolescent with a history of poor frustration management threatens to physically assault one of his teachers, it is the impairment of assaultiveness that is incapacitating and given a severity level of 3. In the course of treatment, one can imagine that the impairment of assaultiveness may be eliminated, but the treatment of the impairment of deficient frustration tolerance may continue for some time. Similarly, if the impairment of pathological grief includes thoughts of suicide, the impairment of suicidal thought/behavior is recorded separately and included in the PIP, and its severity rated separately.

We have identified certain impairments that have the potential on their own to justify more intensive service interventions (e.g., hospitalization). We call these impairments the *critical impairments* (see Table 6-1). We define an impairment as critical when it has the potential to become so severe that it 1) places the safety of the patient or others at risk, or 2) renders the patient significantly dysfunctional in the home or work

---

Table 6–1. Critical impairments

Assaultiveness	Obsessions
Compulsions	Paranoia
Concomitant medical condition	Phobia
Delusions	Psychomotor agitation
Dissociative states	Psychomotor retardation
Dysphoric mood	Psychotic thought and perception
Dysphoric mood with alexithymia	Psychotic thought, perception,
Eating disorder	and behavior
Fire setting	Rage reactions
Hallucinations	Running away
Homicidal thought/behavior	Self-mutilation
Manic thought/behavior	Substance abuse
Mood lability	Suicidal thought/behavior

Note. Critical impairments are those that have the potential on their own to justify more intensive service interventions (e.g., hospitalization).

---

environment. This subgroup of impairments would have level-of-severity ratings from 0 to 4. *Noncritical impairments* have severity ratings from 0 to 2. Although the presence of the noncritical impairments may well impact the treatment of the critical impairments and require their own additional treatment interventions, the noncritical impairments by themselves will not justify the need for the most intensive levels of service. This is a shortcoming of the lengthy patient problem lists that often give reviewers the impression (perhaps a false one) of being devised to "add weight" to the seriousness of the patient's condition and the need for treatment.

It is not the number of impairments but rather the severity level of the critical impairment(s) that influences reviewers. *There is no severity in numbers!* An impairment profile may have only one impairment, but, with sufficient behavioral documentation of the severity level of that impairment, the patient may be justifiably treated at a very intensive level of care.

The impairments we have selected as critical are listed in Table 6-1.

Case Examples

Two patient vignettes are presented below to illustrate the application of behavioral severity levels to the PIP. In the interest of brevity, the discussion of these two cases will focus only on the critical impairments. For each critical impairment identified in the vignettes, we provide a list of patient behaviors that we conceptualize as being individually corroborative for each of the four levels of severity for that particular impairment. After reviewing the clinical data (i.e., patient behaviors) relevant to that patient's impairment, we "match" the behaviors with the defining severity level behaviors in order to determine the appropriate severity level for each impairment.

We will continue to use the case examples of Melanie W. and Bob D. presented in Chapter 5 because they are particularly instructive and illustrative. These cases also will be the clinical examples used in subsequent chapters to illustrate the use of the PIP in determining patient outcome objectives

(Chapter 7), establishing the treatment plan (Chapter 8), and tracking the patient's progress toward meeting those outcome objectives (Chapter 9).

Case 1: Melanie W.

The reader will recall from Chapter 5 that Melanie, believing that she had no future for herself, had verbalized the desire to die. She had stated that she had found an easy way of killing herself: by eating all the sugars she wanted to and not taking her insulin, or by injecting herself with too much insulin. She talked about going to the corner store, buying chocolate bars, and "eating chocolate and getting drunk to have a good time before I die." Melanie fantasized about being in a diabetic coma, dying, with the ambulance arriving minutes too late. She knew the times of the day and locations to go where she would not be found until it was too late. Melanie was habitually truant and spent most of her days at home taking care of her younger siblings, who were largely neglected by both parents.

Patient Impairment Profile   **Patient: Melanie W.**

Critical impairments
1. Suicidal thought/behavior
2. Dysphoric mood with alexithymia
3. Concomitant medical condition (juvenile-type diabetes mellitus)

Noncritical impairments
4. Inadequate health care skills
5. Family dysfunction
6. Truancy

Patient behaviors characterizing/defining severity levels for suicidal thought/behavior:

Severity Level 4: Imminently dangerous
1. Suicidal thought/behavior present daily, placing patient in imminent danger.
2. Suicidal thought/behavior requiring medical or surgical intervention.
3. Past history of dangerous suicide attempts.

Severity Level 3: Incapacitating
1. Suicidal thought/behavior present at least weekly, placing the patient in danger.
2. Recent history of suicide attempts.

Severity Level 2: Debilitating
1. Frequent suicidal ideation present with demonstrable ability to control suicidal behavior.

Severity Level 1: Moderate
1. Suicidal ideation present and verbalized as a problem.

Severity Level 0: Absent, nonpathological
1. No suicidal thought/behavior.

The suicidal thought/behavior in Melanie's impairment profile was assigned a severity level of 4. Melanie's intentional manipulation of her insulin placed her in serious medical danger. Excessive or inadequate insulin administration could be lethal. Her past suicide attempts were very serious and required medical hospitalization to stabilize the brittle, out-of-control diabetic condition in which she presented each time. Her unwillingness to follow her insulin regimen placed her at high risk. One of her past suicide attempts also included cutting both wrists with a razor blade deep enough to necessitate suturing. (After Melanie's referral for a psychiatric evaluation, she was hospitalized in an acute psychiatric unit.)

Patient behaviors characterizing/defining severity levels for dysphoric mood with alexithymia:

Severity Level 4: Imminently dangerous
1. Dysphoric mood renders one totally unable to care for oneself.
2. Ruminations over futility, helplessness, hopelessness, and/or suicide for 75% of the day.
3. Dysphoric mood totally impedes the ability to work or perform complex or varied tasks.
4. Dysphoric mood precludes the ability to maintain attention or concentration for necessary periods of time.
5. Isolation from others severely impedes normative functioning for the greater part of the day.

Severity Level 4: Imminently dangerous (continued)
6. Dysphoric mood obliterates any capacity for pleasure.
7. Dysphoric mood prevents the following of treatment recommendations.

Severity Level 3: Incapacitating
1. Dysphoric mood severely interferes with the carrying out of daily personal, family, work, and financial responsibilities.
2. Ruminations over futility, helplessness, hopelessness, and/or suicide for 50% of the day.
3. Dysphoric mood interferes with ability to maintain attention or concentration for necessary periods of time.
4. Isolation from others affects normative functioning for the greater part of the day.
5. Dysphoric mood leaves patient unable to maintain work pace or perform complex or varied tasks.
6. Dysphoric mood markedly compromises capacity for pleasure.
7. Dysphoric mood interferes with ability to follow treatment recommendations.

Severity Level 2: Debilitating
1. Dysphoric mood impedes adequate completion of activities of daily living.
2. Ruminations over futility, helplessness, hopelessness, and/or suicide for 25% of the day.
3. Dysphoric mood compromises ability to maintain attention and concentration for variable periods of time.
4. Isolation from others affects normative functioning for variable periods of time.
5. Dysphoric mood interrupts work pace or performance of complex or varied tasks.
6. Dysphoric mood diminishes capacity for pleasure.

Severity Level 1: Moderate
1. Dysphoric mood present and verbalized as a problem in daily living.
2. Dysphoric mood affects ability to maintain attention or concentration.
3. Dysphoric mood inclines one to uncomfortable isolation.
4. Dysphoric mood causes distress while patient is functioning at work or performing complex or varied tasks.

Severity Level 0: Absent, nonpathological
1. No evidence of dysphoric mood.

The dysphoric mood with alexithymia in Melanie's impairment profile was assigned a severity level of 4. Melanie's personal hygiene was very poor: dirty hair, unwashed face, and wrinkled and soiled clothes. She verbalized that she did not care how she looked or what others thought of her.

Most of Melanie's statements were self-critical, with expressions of hopelessness and thoughts of suicide. She felt totally helpless in trying to solve her very real family problems, and she was overwhelmed with the self-assigned responsibility of caring for her siblings that she (accurately) felt was necessary, given her parents' deficiencies, ineffectiveness, and unavailability.

Melanie had no desire to attend school and when forced to go was unable to concentrate or complete any assignments. She usually would leave by third period. Melanie often daydreamed, not listening to conversations with teachers or friends, and felt distracted even in her favorite pastime, watching television. She reported a loss of desire to be around people. Being with friends or shopping with her mother no longer was fun. She preferred to hide in her room. The only pleasure she experienced was when intoxicated by alcohol. Melanie also verbalized that she did not have the energy or the desire to try any of the suggestions made by family, friends, medical doctors, or therapists. Her answer "Why bother!" had ceased to be a question.

Patient behaviors characterizing/defining severity levels for a concomitant medical condition:

Severity Level 4: Imminently dangerous
1. Medical condition life-threatening to the patient, requiring acute stabilization.
2. Medical condition severely interferes with taking physical care of oneself.
3. Totally unwilling to follow prescribed medical treatment regimen for a potentially life-threatening condition.
4. Total denial of the condition and its ramifications.

Severity Level 3: Incapacitating
1. Medical condition dangerous but not imminently life-threatening to the patient.
2. Unwilling to agree to follow prescribed medical treatment regimen.
3. Requires medical-surgical intervention not available as an outpatient.
4. Medical condition markedly compromises (greater than 50%) taking physical care of oneself.
5. Denial of the medical condition and its ramifications present.

Severity Level 2: Debilitating
1. Medical condition unstable.
2. Medical condition compromises (greater than 25%) taking physical care of oneself.
3. Patient agrees with, but does not subsequently demonstrate adherence to, the prescribed medical treatment regimen.

Severity Level 1: Moderate
1. Medical condition present but does not require daily medical supervision.
2. Evidence of adherence to a prescribed treatment regimen in the presence of ongoing support or monitoring.
3. Verbalized unresolved concerns regarding the medical condition and its ramifications.

Severity Level 0: Absent, nonpathological
1. Medical condition under control or no longer present.
2. Patient accepts the presence and ramifications of the medical condition and adheres to the prescribed treatment independently.

Initially, the concomitant medical condition in Melanie's impairment profile was assigned a severity level of 4. Without proper medical management, Melanie was at critical risk for a number of the life-threatening complications of untreated diabetes mellitus. She required acute medical care (hospitalization) in order to be stabilized. Melanie had been refusing to monitor her blood glucose levels prior to hospitalization, and, although she was well educated as to how to do so, her overall management of her diabetes was very poor.

Melanie's PIP with initial severity level ratings is summarily presented as follows:

Patient Impairment Profile	Patient: Melanie W.
	Severity
Critical impairments	
1. Suicidal thought/behavior	4
2. Dysphoric mood with alexithymia	4
3. Concomitant medical condition (juvenile-type diabetes mellitus)	4
Noncritical impairments	
4. Inadequate health care skills	2
5. Family dysfunction	2
6. Truancy	2

Case 2: Bob D.

Bob's clinical presentation was detailed in Chapter 5 and will only be summarized here. Bob, a 23-year-old white married male, was brought to an emergency room by his parents for an acute episode of delusional behavior and acute alcohol intoxication. Bob presented with bizarre religious delusions that he felt gave him the right and power to break into buildings, claim them as God's, and then demolish them in order to appropriate the land for children's parks. Married for just over a year, Bob had never settled into a job in which he felt comfortable. He had been observed on many occasions to be a volatile, at times verbally explosive man with a severely compromised ability to manage day-to-day stressors.

Patient Impairment Profile	Patient: Bob D.
Critical impairments	
1. Delusions	
2. Substance abuse (alcohol)	
Noncritical impairment	
3. Deficient frustration tolerance	

Patient behaviors characterizing/defining severity levels for delusions:

Severity Level 4: Imminently dangerous
1. Daily preoccupation with delusions, placing patient or others in imminent danger.
2. Delusions totally interfere with ability to care for oneself.
3. Delusions totally interfere with ability to follow treatment recommendations.
4. Delusions totally interfere with ability to work or perform complex or varied tasks.
5. Delusions preclude the ability to maintain attention or concentration for necessary periods of time.

Severity Level 3: Incapacitating
1. Preoccupation with the delusions, placing patient or others in danger.
2. Delusions interfere with carrying out personal, family, work, and/or financial responsibilities.
3. Delusions interfere with ability to follow treatment recommendations.
4. Delusions interfere with ability to maintain adequate work pace or perform most complex or varied tasks.
5. Delusions interfere with ability to maintain attention or concentration for necessary periods of time.

Severity Level 2: Debilitating
1. Delusions disruptive to the daily functioning of self or others.
2. Delusions interrupt work pace or performance of complex or varied tasks.
3. Delusions interfere with ability to maintain attention or concentration for variable periods of time.

Severity Level One: Moderate
1. Delusions prevent normative, optimal daily functioning.
2. Delusions compromise optimal work pace or the performance of complex and varied tasks.
3. Delusions compromise the capacity to maintain optimal attention or concentration.

Severity Level 0: Absent, nonpathological
1. No delusions present.

The delusions in Bob's impairment profile were assigned a severity level of 4. The delusions confirmed his right to break into buildings, placing him (and perhaps others) in imminent danger. In this regard, he demonstrated a total absence of judgment and was unable to care for himself. He was at times too preoccupied with his own delusional beliefs to listen accurately or to concentrate, let alone follow any treatment recommendations or perform any complex or varied tasks. (Bob was in fact admitted to the intensive care unit of a psychiatric hospital.)

Patient behaviors characterizing/defining severity levels for substance abuse:

Severity Level 4: Imminently dangerous
1. Substance abuse present daily, placing patient or others in imminent danger.
2. Complete denial of the substance abuse and its ramifications.
3. Substance abuse totally interferes with the ability to care for oneself.
4. Cessation of abused substance would precipitate a life-threatening physical withdrawal requiring close medical attention.
5. Substance abuse totally interferes with the ability to maintain work pace or perform complex or varied tasks.
6. Substance abuse precludes the ability to maintain attention or concentration for necessary periods of time.

Severity Level 3: Incapacitating
1. Substance abuse present daily or weekly, placing patient or others in danger.
2. The uncontrollable urge to abuse is present daily.
3. Denial of the substance abuse and its ramifications.
4. Profound psychological dependence present.
5. Substance abuse interferes with carrying out daily personal, family, work, and financial responsibilities.
6. Substance abuse interferes with ability to follow treatment recommendations.
7. Substance abuse interferes with ability to maintain work pace or perform complex or varied tasks.
8. Substance abuse interferes with ability to maintain attention or concentration for necessary periods of time.

Severity Level 2: Debilitating
1. Substance abuse disrupts daily functioning of self or others.
2. Uncontrollable urge to abuse is present weekly.
3. Denial of one or more aspects of the substance abuse.
4. Substance abuse interrupts work pace or performance of complex and varied tasks.
5. Substance abuse interferes with ability to maintain concentration for variable periods of time.

Severity Level 1: Moderate
1. Substance abuse prevents normative, optimal daily functioning.
2. Substance abuse is present and verbalized as a problem.
3. Urge to abuse is present weekly.
4. Substance abuse compromises optimal work pace and performance of complex and varied tasks.
5. Substance abuse compromises capacity to maintain optimal attention or concentration.

Severity Level 0: Absent, nonpathological
1. No substance abuse.

The substance abuse (alcohol) in Bob's impairment profile was assigned a severity level of 4 at the time of admission. The question was raised as to whether the delusional disorder was the result of alcohol or some other drug intoxication. Regardless of the cause, however, the delusions placed Bob in imminent danger because of their content. With a reported daily intake of six to eight beers, the possibility of his drinking much more than that and the possibility of his having a life-threatening physical withdrawal were active treatment concerns. Certainly at the time of admission, Bob was totally unable to take care of himself. Bob's initial PIP with initial severity level ratings is summarily presented as follows:

Patient Impairment Profile	Patient: Bob D.
	Severity
Critical impairments	
1. Delusions	4
2. Substance abuse (alcohol)	4
Noncritical impairment	
3. Deficient frustration tolerance	2

On the second day of hospitalization, it was established that Bob had actually been experiencing a phencyclidine- (or PCP) induced delusional disorder. By that time, the delusional disorder had run its course, and there was no evidence of alcohol withdrawal thus far. No further evidence could be found to establish an alcohol intake of more than the six beers a day reported earlier. The adjustment of severity levels as treatment proceeds—and the usefulness of tracking severity ratings as one way of measuring and articulating the patient's progress in treatment—will be addressed in Chapter 9.

Conclusion

The assignment of severity level ratings is a convenient, shorthand method for documenting and graphically summarizing the seriousness of the patient's PIP. When we refer to "communication" with external reviewers, we are simultaneously proposing that the PIP and the severity level ratings can be used to organize the treatment documentation in the medical record. It makes sense that the medical record should contain the information that external reviewers need to know, especially if or when the external review process does, in fact, return to the medical record for the clinical information necessary to make reimbursement decisions. This method of recording information is in the interest of the patient, the practitioner, and the reviewer. More will be said about treatment documentation in Chapters 9 and 10, wherein we offer a model that satisfies the multiple documentation requirements that mental healthcare practitioners and facilities are currently expected to meet.

When talking on the telephone with a reviewer about the seriousness of the patient's impairments, we present the PIP and describe each impairment by its severity (i.e., imminently dangerous, incapacitating, debilitating, or moderate), and offer two or three patient behaviors or patient statements that corroborate that severity level rating. This is the clinical information reviewers need to know in order to justify a particular intensity of service.

During the initial contact with the reviewer, more information is usually requested from the practitioner—for example, the goals and objectives, the treatment plan, and the estimated length of stay or duration of treatment. How the practitioner responds to these questions is the subject of the next two chapters.

Chapter 7

Patient Outcome Objectives

"What are the goals and objectives?"

The authors review the confusing and inconsistent use of the terms "goal" and "objective" and suggest adherence to clinical outcome as a measure of treatment progress and clinical effectiveness. Outcome objectives are met by the patient, not the practitioner. Individualized behavioral patient outcome objectives are identified for each impairment in the Patient Impairment Profile, consistent with both the severity of the impairments and the patient's strengths and limitations. Critical impairments (i.e., those that can be assigned a severity rating of 3 or 4) have defined patient outcome objectives that are to be met by the time of discharge from an acute treatment setting. After an impairment is no longer critical, new outcome objectives are defined for the impairment(s) that are to be met by the end of treatment.

W e will now discuss how the Patient Impairment Profile (PIP) links the determination of severity to the development of patient outcome objectives that comply with Joint Commission and Medicare guidelines for treatment plan documentation. This approach is valuable for the practitioner and the facility because external reviewers currently request the same assessment and treatment planning information that the Joint Commission requires for accreditation.

The determination of the severity of the patient's impairment(s) and the subsequent decision about the appropriate level of care (i.e., outpatient, partial hospitalization, inpatient, or intensive inpatient) are based upon evaluation of all the facts available during the initial contact with the patient, which is usually at a time of crisis. During this "intake process," the presenting complaints, history of the present illness, and family, social, and medical histories are obtained; a mental status examination is performed; the results of a DSM-III-R multiaxial evaluation are recorded; and the concerns (impairments) to be addressed in treatment are specified (the PIP) and rated as to their severity. For patients requiring treatment in an accredited residential facility or hospital, this data set comprises the "initial assessment" and is the groundwork for developing the "preliminary treatment plan."

As soon as possible thereafter, the clinician or a member of the treatment team has the responsibility to perform and document a "complete assessment" and develop a written and comprehensive "individualized treatment plan" based on the patient's clinical needs. The terms "initial assessment," "preliminary treatment plan," "complete assessment," and "individualized treatment plan" are specifically referenced in the *Consolidated Standards Manual* (CSM) (Joint Commission 1990a).[1] The CSM contains detailed standards of care for

---

[1]Even though most psychiatric hospitals are now surveyed for accreditation by the Joint Commission utilizing the *Accreditation Manual for Hospitals* (AMH) (Joint Commission 1991), it is the detail of the CSM that still provides administrators and practitioners servicing mental healthcare facilities with the content for policy and procedure manuals, assessment forms, and treatment plans.

organizations providing mental health services, substance abuse services, and services for mentally retarded and developmentally disabled persons. The patient evaluation process, the type of detailed information that comprises a complete assessment and treatment plan, and time frames for completion are spelled out in the CSM.

The patient's particular impairment profile addresses "the complete assessment" required in the 1991 CSM (Standard PM.11.1), in that it does summarily identify the "physical, emotional, behavioral, social, recreational, and, when appropriate, legal, vocational, and nutritional needs" of the patient. Note that there is no requirement for a "problem list." In fact, the term is not even mentioned in the CSM. The PIP identifies, in behavioral terms, those issues that require, and can benefit from, treatment. It also clarifies which impairments, based on their severity rating, require a more intensive level of care.

It is axiomatic that treatment plans include "goals" and "objectives." And yet, an informal review of hundreds of individual practitioner and multidisciplinary treatment plans reveals a conspicuous absence of congruency in the understanding and employment of these two terms. At times they are used interchangeably or blended together (e.g., "resolution of marital conflict"); at other times they are descriptors of endpoints for the patient to meet (e.g., "improved communication with spouse"); and, not infrequently, they are described as targets at which the practitioner is aiming (e.g., "teach active listening skills").

The 1991 CSM offers clarification on this point. Standard PM.27 requires that the treatment plan contain "specific goals that the patient must achieve to attain, maintain, and/or reestablish emotional and/or physical health as well as maximum growth and adaptive capabilities." Note the emphasis on the fact that the goals are the patient's, not the practitioner's. Standard PM.28 states that the treatment plan must also contain "specific objectives that relate to the goals [as defined by Standard PM.27], are written in measurable terms, and include expected achievement dates." The specific objectives are also those of the patient, not the practitioner. The clarity of terms offered by the CSM, however, becomes muddied when juxtaposed with federal guidelines and individual state regulations with which practitioners must also comply.

Medicare guidelines call for both "long-range and short-range goals" but do not define those terms (Federal Register, January 3, 1984, pp. 315–316). The distinction between the long-range and short-range goals of the federal guidelines is, we feel, a confusing and difficult one to make. Short-range goals appear to be guideposts representing intermediate time spans during care. A series of short-range goals, when met, should achieve a final, accomplishable, desirable result. The last short-range goal might well be the final one and would have been called the long-range goal if set at the beginning of the series! Short-range goals may be useful ongoing clinical tools, but only a long-range goal carries the connotation of outcome for an episode of care (Grant 1981). The AMH and CSM no longer distinguish between long-range and short-range treatment goals.

If this were not bewildering enough, some states, such as Colorado, also require that the treatment plan contain "goals that are measurable and have identified target dates for their completion" (Grant 1981). A "goal" in Colorado very closely approximates an "objective" for the Joint Commission. The term "measurable" carries the explicit need for some form of quantification—a task for which most mental healthcare practitioners have never been adequately trained. And which goals are to be measured? The short-range goals? The long-range goals? Both? The 1991 CSM (Standard PM.27) implies that the completion of treatment goals occurs when the patient has "attain[ed] . . . maximum growth and adaptive capabilities,"— that is, the completion of treatment. Actual achievement dates are assigned only to the patient's measurable objectives.

Returning to the language of impairments, we define the goal(s) of treatment as the amelioration or "repair" of the identified impairments in the PIP. Goal achievement as stated in the 1991 CSM is expressed in the language of impairments by the repair of the impairment profile: the patient is returned to maximum wellness ("maximum growth and adaptive capabilities") (Standard PM.27). Of course, the optimal goal for a patient is the absence of any impairment. At the time of assessment, we tend to "set our sights high" and anticipate that the patient's impairments can be eliminated. However, a patient's limitations or deficiencies may make the attainment of such a goal not possible. The patient's goal(s) for each impairment must then be reevaluated and adjusted, when necessary, to reasonably achievable levels. For example, some patients with the impairment of paranoia may never be free from persecutory or jealous delusional beliefs; however, reducing the disabling intensity of those beliefs with the proper medication might be an achievable goal.

During the initial telephone contact with an outside reviewer, questions are typically asked regarding the "treatment plan," the "goals" and "objectives," and the estimated length of treatment. Using the impairment model, we respond by providing the reviewer with specific patient outcome objectives selected for each impairment in the profile, based upon the patient's strengths/limitations. We indicate that the patient's outcome objectives are expected to be met by the completion of the particular level of treatment we are recommending.

In a "vertically integrated" system of mental healthcare services, there are multiple levels of treatment services available (e.g., intensive inpatient care, partial hospitalization, day treatment services, intensive outpatient treatment, medication management). Except when the patient is being treated at the lowest level of care (upon completion of which the patient is supposed to be well), the patient's outcome objectives are designed to be met at the time of completion of a particular level of care. From that point, the patient moves on to continued treatment at a lower level of care with new patient outcome objectives for each impairment specific for that level. The estimated length of time it will take for the patient to meet these objectives is the answer to the reviewer's question regarding the "length of stay" (at a particular level of care) or "duration of treatment" (completion of the lowest level of care). The only target dates that we specify are those for meeting the patient outcome objectives of each impairment. The date of completion of repair of the last remaining impairment (to whatever degree possible) is the duration of treatment.

Case Examples

In the two clinical vignettes presented below, we will include the initial patient outcome objectives that we determined for both patients' impairments at the time of the initial assessment. Characteristically, they are "set high," pending further assessment of the patient's strengths and limitations. In the case of Bob D., his initial impairment profile changed significantly by the third day of hospitalization when the multidisciplinary treatment plan was written. The integration of the assessments and observational data in this case required that the profile be updated to accurately reflect the evolving dynamic understanding of the case. Patient outcome objectives would be reevaluated and changed as well. (The consensually agreed-upon PIP that resulted and the revised outcome objectives are included in the description of the development of Bob's multidisciplinary treatment plan in Chapter 8.)

The outcome objectives of the critical impairments (those with severity ratings of three or four) are expected to be met by the time of the patient's discharge from the acute treatment setting. The objectives for the noncritical impairments are expected to be met by the end of treatment. These latter outcome objectives are not included as the primary evidence for the more acute level of care (i.e., hospitalization) that the patients received. This notwithstanding, the presence of noncritical impairments may significantly impact the treatment of the critical ones and may well be the supportive evidence that documents why the patient's progress toward meeting the outcome objectives may be delayed.

Case 1: Melanie W.

Patient Impairment Profile   **Patient: Melanie W.**

10/3   **Severity**

Critical impairments

1.	Suicidal thought/behavior	4
2.	Dysphoric mood with alexithymia	4
3.	Concomitant medical condition (juvenile-type diabetes mellitus)	4

Patient Impairment Profile   **Patient: Melanie W.**

10/3   **Severity**

(continued)

Noncritical impairments

4.	Inadequate health care skills	2
5.	Family dysfunction	2
6.	Truancy	2

Patient Outcome Objectives

(To be met by 11/3—estimated discharge date)

Delusions

1. Patient will demonstrate a 50% improvement in the SAAD Scale (rated at the time of admission) within 72 hours.
2. Patient will eliminate active suicidal thoughts/behavior within 72 hours as demonstrated by the absence of communications (verbal or behavioral) about planning or wanting to die.
3. Patient will eliminate active suicidal thoughts/intentions within 72 hours as evidenced by statements that she has no plans or wishes to die.
4. Patient will verbalize the precipitant(s) of suicidal thoughts/behaviors to staff and therapist.
5. Patient will verbalize to staff and therapist what alternative actions will be implemented if feeling suicidal in the future.
6. Patient will complete and present to staff and therapist a discharge plan form that includes outpatient follow-up appointments, a contingency plan of action should the suicidal ideation return, and, if applicable, the medication regimen to be followed.

Dysphoric mood with alexithymia

1. Patient will acknowledge awareness of changes in mood as demonstrated by patient reports to staff and therapist.
2. Patient will demonstrate recognition of precipitating factors for negative mood changes and seek help from a staff member or therapist accordingly.
3. Patient will demonstrate reduction in the dysphoric mood as evidenced at the time of discharge by a 50% decrease in the Hamilton Depression Rating Scale (rated at the initiation of treatment).

4. Patient's dysphoric mood will be lessened as demonstrated by staff observations of:
   a. Increased self-directed initiation of activities—within 1 week.
   b. Elimination of isolative activities—within 1 week.
   c. Increased integrating behaviors with others in the treatment setting—within 2 weeks.
   d. Verbalization of plans to be initiated with family members or friends—within 3 weeks.
   e. Pairing up with a newer patient in the treatment program and helping this patient integrate into the treatment program within 3 weeks.
5. Patient will demonstrate a reduction in dysphoric mood as evidenced by a change from negative, self-deprecating statements to positive hopeful statements about self and life—measured by a 50% improvement in the Coopersmith Self-Esteem Inventory and evidenced by statements to staff and therapist.
6. Patient will complete and present to staff and therapist a discharge plan form that includes outpatient follow-up appointments, a contingency plan of action should the dysphoric mood intensify, and, if applicable, the medication regimen to be followed.
7. The patient will be able to distinguish between pleasurable and unpleasurable affects and label one of each of them accordingly.

**Concomitant medical condition
(juvenile-type diabetes mellitus)**

1. Patient will verbalize thoughts and feelings regarding the medical condition to at least one staff member within 24 hours.
2. Patient will be aware of the concomitant medical condition as measured by completion of a self-care worksheet that describes the condition, its etiology, prognosis, treatment regimen, and potential and possible future complications.
3. Patient will demonstrate awareness and understanding of the medical condition by active compliance with the treatment regimen (e.g., self-initiated medication compliance, self-selected appropriate diet).
4. Patient will complete and present to staff and therapist a discharge plan form that specifies outpatient follow-up psychotherapy appointments; medical follow-up visits; names and phone numbers of physicians treating the condition; emergency phone numbers and hospital names, addresses, and phone numbers; a contingency plan of action should the medical condition worsen; and the medical treatment regimen for the condition to be followed.

Patient Outcome Objectives

(To be met by the end of treatment—estimate 2/1)

Inadequate health care skills

1. Patient will improve health care skills as demonstrated by bathing, brushing teeth, combing hair, and wearing clean clothes daily.
2. Patient will improve health care skills as demonstrated by selecting nutritious foods from the four food groups at mealtime as observed by staff and/or therapist.
3. Patient will demonstrate the ability to manage future health care as demonstrated by a written health care plan specifying medical visits, names and numbers of physicians, emergency phone numbers, and a dental care plan.

Family dysfunction

1. Patient will articulate awareness of her dysfunctional role within the family to staff and therapist.
2. Patient will articulate to staff and therapist her past role within the family and a plan for modifying that role.
3. Patient will articulate to staff and therapist the warning signs of renewed family dysfunction that require emergency outside help.
4. Patient will demonstrate improved understanding and amelioration of the family dysfunction as evidenced by:
    a. Discussion among family members as to what their dysfunctional roles were.
    b. Written clarification in family therapy of the "non-negotiables" for each family member.
    c. Development of a written family contract that specifies what the plans for change in the family dysfunction will be and what plan of action will be taken when significant disagreement occurs.
5. Patient will complete and present to staff and therapist a discharge plan containing a) follow-up family therapy, including the specification of warning signs for more intensive treatment; or b) placement.

Truancy

1. Patient will acknowledge the problem of truancy as demonstrated by a written paper that identifies the precipitating factors for the truancy and the adverse consequences for being truant.
2. Patient will negotiate a written contract with the family regarding the consequences of continued truancy.
3. Patient will meet with an educator/counselor and develop a written contract for repairing the specific educational deficits resulting from truancy.

Melanie's initial clinical presentation did not change or fluctuate very much in the first 2 weeks of her hospitalization. As a result, the outcome objectives selected for her in the initial assessment remained unchanged throughout her hospitalization.

Case 2: Bob D.

Patient Impairment Profile   Patient: Bob D.

9/1   **Severity**

Critical impairments

1. Delusions   4
2. Substance abuse (alcohol)   4

Noncritical impairments

3. Deficient frustration tolerance   2

Patient Outcome Objectives

(To be met by 9/22)

Delusions

1. Patient will verbalize awareness of the delusional thinking as demonstrated by reports to staff and therapist.
2. Patient will be free of delusions for 72 hours as demonstrated by patient, staff, and therapist report.
3. Patient will verbalize the precipitant(s) of the delusional thinking to staff and therapist.
4. Patient will demonstrate compliance with the medical treatment of the delusions.
5. Patient will complete and present to staff and therapist a discharge plan form that includes outpatient follow-up appointments, a contingency plan of action should the delusions recur, and the medication regimen to be followed.

Substance abuse (alcohol)

1. Patient will demonstrate understanding of the disease process of substance abuse as measured by the completion of a written "step 1" that satisfactorily records the adverse impact of the abuse on the patient's life.

Patient Outcome Objectives (continued)

(To be met by 9/22)

Substance abuse (alcohol) (continued)

2. Patient will demonstrate understanding of the disease process of substance abuse as demonstrated by a three- to five-page paper that addresses substance abuse as a disease, the problem of substance-substitution abuse, relapse indicators, and relapse avoidance techniques.
3. Patient will present at a 12-step meeting and/or to a newcomer in the treatment setting the adverse impact of the substance abuse and potential hazards of substance-substitution abuse.
4. Patient will demonstrate absence of substance abuse during treatment as evidenced by negative, random urine drug screenings.
5. Patient will have one pass with a subsequent clean urine drug screen prior to discharge.
6. Patient will be able to specify to staff and therapist a plan of action to be implemented when there is an urge to use again.
7. Patient will maintain sobriety as demonstrated by a written personal aftercare plan that includes a minimum of four aftercare meetings, three to four outside support groups a week (including names and locations), and outpatient psychotherapy.
8. Patient will successfully implement the written personal aftercare plan for 1 week within the current treatment setting.
9. Patient will obtain a 12-step (interim) sponsor and introduce the sponsor to the primary therapist.

Patient Outcome Objectives

(To be met by the end of treatment—estimate 1/11)

Deficient frustration tolerance

1. Patient will acknowledge awareness of the deficient frustration tolerance as measured by a report to staff of at least one situation in which the low tolerance resulted in a confrontational episode.
2. Patient will acknowledge understanding of the deficient frustration tolerance as demonstrated by a written paper on how it has affected the patient's life, what situations provoke adverse responses, and how these situations might be handled differently.
3. Patient will take positive action to mitigate a heretofore frustrating situation as observed by or reported to staff and therapist.

Conclusion

Both of these patients' hospital stays were subject to concurrent external review that monitored the clinical necessity for continued inpatient treatment. Patient outcome objectives structure our thinking for documenting the clinical rationale for treatment, and they simplify the task of communicating both the rationale for continued treatment and the patient's progress (see Chapter 9). We always refer to the outcome objectives when talking with outside reviewers. We utilize the objectives to resolve the disturbing dilemma that all practitioners face when seeking continued authorization for treatment services (at every level of care): practitioners must communicate that the treatment plan is working (i.e., the patient is getting better) and at the same time convey to the reviewer that the patient requires additional treatment at that level of care (i.e., the patient is still sick). Documented behavioral statements such as "Melanie is smiling more and attending her activities without prompting" communicate the progress and effectiveness of the treatment. When the practitioner also provides behavioral evidence that the patient is still at risk—for example, "Melanie returned to her room in tears after she exploded in a family session with her mother and father; she then told a nurse that 'I was right all along. Nothing's ever going to change. Things are hopeless.'"—a case is also being made and substantiated by the patient's behaviors that Melanie is not ready to return home.

A format for documenting this treatment information in the medical record, corroborating and substantiating the ongoing modification of the multidisciplinary treatment plan, is presented in Chapter 9. Chapter 8 addresses another necessary component of the treatment plan: the practitioners' treatment interventions. Like the severity ratings and outcome objectives, the specification of treatment interventions can also be guided and organized by the PIP.

Chapter 8

Treatment Interventions
and the Treatment Plan

"How are you planning to treat the patient?"

The patient's treatment plan should include the patient impairment profile (PIP) and severity ratings, identified patient outcome objectives, and treatment interventions for each impairment. In this chapter we describe how the PIP structures the selection of treatment interventions by each modality and links them to both the impairments and the patient outcome objectives. Two case vignettes illustrate the selection of treatment interventions based upon the PIP.

I n our experience, all outside reviewers request information regarding the "treatment plan." Some ask for it early in the discussion without inquiring about "goals and objectives"; other reviewers ask for goals and objectives when, in fact, they want to know what we are going to be doing for the patient; still other reviewers ask for both. Whenever possible, we take the initiative to offer a reviewer the evaluation and treatment information in the order detailed in this book: the patient impairment profile (PIP), the severity of the impairments, the patient's outcome objectives with anticipated target dates for their completion, and, as described in this chapter, the treatment interventions.

External reviewers appear to utilize a variety of operational definitions for goals, objectives, and treatment plan. We tried to clarify the meaning of the terms "goals" and "objectives" in Chapter 7. There is also considerable confusion about the difference between a plan and a goal—and this lack of clear use of this terminology is not limited to reviewers. In an interesting study conducted at a workshop on record keeping, a group of statements was presented to clinicians who were then asked to decide whether each statement was a plan or a goal. Opinion was split almost evenly on both choices (Grant 1981).

For instance, "Start the patient on lithium carbonate" and "Teach assertiveness skills" are ambiguous. Considering the first example as a plan, the goal may have been normalization of the manic episode. On the other hand, ensuring that the patient takes lithium could be a goal, and the plan may have been to ameliorate the problem of reluctance to take medications, using verbal persuasion. Likewise, teaching assertiveness skills may be a plan to meet the goal to increase assertiveness. It may also function as a goal when addressing inadequate survival skills with a patient who may be lacking in this area. In each case, whether the statement is a goal or a plan depends on knowing how the problem was formulated and whether the person making the statement intended it to be a goal or a plan.

This ambiguity has been a considerable source of difficulty in helping clinicians meet guidelines for explicit treatment planning. The standard dictionary (*Webster's New World*) definition of a plan as "a formulated scheme for getting something done" is different from what federal guidelines and the 1991

CSM respectively call a "multidisciplinary" or "individualized" treatment plan. Under the heading "Treatment Plan" in the federal guidelines is a parenthesis containing "clinical evaluation of patient status on admission, prescribed treatment, treatment given, and long- and short-term goals." The CSM is similar except that it changes the order of the components (identification of goals and objectives comes before specification of treatment interventions) and clearly states that the treatment plan must contain "specific goals" that the *patient* must attain (PM.27), "specific, measurable objectives" that the *patient* will achieve (PM.28), and a description of "the services, activities, and programs planned for the patient and the staff members assigned to work with the patient" (PM.29).

A dictionary of treatment interventions for the impairments that we devised for the specific treatment modality of individual psychotherapy is given in Appendix B. As explained in Chapter 3, a variety of mental healthcare professionals may implement the interventions used in a single treatment modality. In California, psychiatrists, clinical psychologists, clinical social workers, and marriage, family, and child counselors may all offer individual psychotherapy and bill for their services using the same "Current Procedural Terminology" (CPT) code (American Medical Association 1991). Each of these types of practitioners is now also subject to outside review prior to being reimbursed by third-party payers. A practitioner may also elect to treat a patient with more than one modality (e.g., individual psychotherapy and biofeedback) and bill for these services separately using each of their respective procedure codes. Each treatment modality may, of course, be subject to the same external review as well. For these reasons, we prefer to categorize and document therapeutic treatment interventions by modality employed rather than by discipline or clinical specialty.

At more intensive levels of care, a substantial number of treatment modalities may be used to impact the PIP. Practitioners will implement interventions that are specific to the particular modality being used and appropriate for their level of training and clinical expertise. Typically, a hospitalized psychiatric patient will receive nursing services and individual psychotherapy, as well as a combination of other modalities such as group psychotherapy, individual family therapy, psychodrama, biofeedback, assertiveness training, leisure-time skills planning, dietary counseling, and so on. Each treatment modality does not necessarily treat every impairment in a patient's profile.

The 1991 CSM states that the medical record must include "all treatment rendered to the patient" (PM.34.12). Different modalities may be effective in having a beneficial impact on different impairments. The nursing staff, attending clinician, and/or primary therapist typically address each impairment in the PIP from their own particular vantage point. Some treatment modalities may only be of benefit for certain impairments. For example, biofeedback may be very successfully applied to the impairments of rage reactions or psychomotor agitation and only be of limited value in treating delusions or dissociative states. A dictionary of treatment interventions for all the Impairments that are addressed by each treatment modality is beyond the scope of this book. We have included our interpretation of the different therapeutic treatment interventions employed in individual psychotherapy for each of the Impairments (see Appendix B). Hopefully, these interventions can serve as models for practitioners employing other treatment modalities.

The interventions for each impairment in the dictionary in Appendix B are listed in chronological order whenever possible. The interventions that the practitioner typically implements earliest in a course of treatment with individual psychotherapy are listed first because they are usually the first ones selected for inclusion in the preliminary treatment plan generated at the time of the initial assessment. As the treatment progresses, it may be decided that specific individual psychotherapy interventions are completed or that they need to be deleted, substituted, or added. Whenever a decision is made about a particular intervention, we retain that intervention on the updated treatment plan, set it apart by running a dash line through it, and record the decision made for that intervention plus the date in parentheses.

We do not recommend that practitioners itemize in their initial treatment plan everything they *might* choose to do in the future. Like the number of impairments in a profile, this is another case where "more is less." Until all the clinical assessment data are gathered, reviewed, and synthesized, it may not be clear, for example, whether a trial on antidepressant medication is warranted for a suicidal patient.

For some of the impairments, the individual psychotherapy intervention "Assess for the presence of other impairments" may be selected. Because the PIP is designed to be a "living document" that reflects the increased understanding of the nature of the patient's difficulties, what was initially assessed as an impairment (e.g., decreased concentration) may come to be understood as only a symptom of a dysphoric mood that did not behaviorally manifest itself during the initial contact. It is our practice to then update the PIP to reflect the change from decreased concentration to dysphoric mood. The reader is reminded that, though the practitioner may speculate that the patient "must be depressed," until there is concrete behavioral evidence sufficient to document that speculation, the impairment of dysphoric mood is not included in the profile. In this case, it is usually sufficient to provide a reviewer with the behavioral examples of the impairment known to be present while investigation proceeds to establish an explanation (and, typically, a subsequently more accurate descriptor) for the decreased concentration.

Case Examples

We return to the cases of Melanie and Bob and present the interventions selected by the practitioner who both evaluated these patients and performed the individual psychotherapy. A dictionary of individual psychotherapy interventions for each of the impairments that may be evaluated as *critical* (severity rating Level 3 or 4) is located in Appendix B. Once again, this dictionary is neither definitive nor exhaustive. Other practitioners may employ different interventions to impact these impairments, and they are encouraged to specify them in their own treatment plans. All the interventions listed for each Impairment are not necessarily appropriate for every patient. In some cases where several impairments in one patient's profile contain the same interventions (e.g., "Assess the need for evaluation by specific support services" or "Establish a therapeutic alliance"), it is not necessary to restate the intervention every time. At other times, interventions such as "Clarify/interpret the dynamics of [the impairment]" should be repeated for each impairment for which the techniques of clarification or interpretation are planned to be used. The more interventions the practitioner documents—with subsequent behavioral data validating their effectiveness—the more information is available for monitoring clinical competence.

Case 1: Melanie W.

Initial Treatment Plan (10/3)

Patient Impairment Profile   Melanie W.

                                                             Severity

Critical impairments

1. Suicidal thought/behavior   4
2. Dysphoric mood with alexithymia   4
3. Concomitant medical condition
     (juvenile-type diabetes mellitus)   4

Noncritical impairments

1. Inadequate health care skills   2
2. Family dysfunction   2
3. Truancy   2

Patient Outcome Objectives

See Chapter 6 for complete listing of outcome objectives for Melanie W.

Treatment Interventions

Suicidal thought/behavior

Individual psychotherapy
1. Assess the need for evaluation by specific support services: psychological testing, social services, activities therapy, psychodrama.

Suicidal thought/behavior (continued)

Individual psychotherapy (continued)
2. Establish a therapeutic alliance.
3. Assess the lethality of the suicidal thought/behavior and the need for a contained environment for the patient's safety.
4. Identify the precipitants for the suicidal thought/behavior.

Dysphoric mood with alexithymia

Individual psychotherapy
1. Identify the nature/extent of the dysphoric mood with alexithymia.
2. Evaluate for treatment with psychopharmacological agents.
3. Encourage the patient's exploration and verbalization of the issues contributing to the dysphoric mood.
4. Help the patient identify behavioral or somatic equivalents of affective expression.

Concomitant medical condition (juvenile-type diabetes mellitus)

Individual psychotherapy
1. Obtain an accurate assessment and appropriate medical treatment for the condition (including prognosis).
2. Encourage the patient's accurate understanding of the limitations and restrictions imposed by the medical illness.
3. Explore and encourage ventilation of the patient's thoughts and feelings about the medical illness.

Inadequate health care skills

Individual psychotherapy
1. Identify the specific areas of inadequate health care skills.
2. Identify the cause of inadequate health care skills.

Family dysfunction

Individual psychotherapy
1. Identify the nature of the family dysfunction.
2. Support the patient's participation in family therapy to ameliorate the family dysfunction.

Truancy

Individual psychotherapy
1. Identify the nature and extent of the truancy.
2. Identify the educational impact of the truancy.
3. Identify other impairments (e.g., learning disability) contributing to the truancy.

Case 2: Bob D.

Initial Treatment Plan (9/1)

Patient Impairment Profile   **Bob D.**

                                                                  Severity

Critical impairments

1. Delusions   4
2. Substance abuse (alcohol)   4

Noncritical impairments

3. Deficient frustration tolerance   2

Patient Outcome Objectives

See Chapter 6 for complete listing of outcome objectives for Bob D.

Treatment Interventions

Delusions

Individual psychotherapy
1. Assess the need for evaluation by specific support services: psychological testing, social services, substance abuse counseling, activities therapy.
2. Establish a therapeutic alliance.
3. Identify the nature and etiology of the delusions.
4. Rule out the presence of a concomitant medical condition as etiologic for the delusions.
5. Evaluate the delusions for psychopharmacological treatment.
6. Treat the delusions with psychopharmacological agents.

Substance abuse

Individual psychotherapy
1. Obtain a definitive history of the nature and extent of the substance abuse.
2. Implement a random urine drug screening plan.

Deficient frustration tolerance

Individual psychotherapy
1. Identify the triggers and current threshold of deficient frustration tolerance.
2. Rule out the presence of concomitant impairments.

Conclusion

The PIP, with patient outcome objectives and treatment interventions, comprises an initial treatment plan that is more lengthy and time-consuming to generate than practitioners are generally accustomed to doing. However, the time-saving benefits of such efforts are to be found in updating the treatment plan, documenting the patient's progress as treatment proceeds, writing the discharge summary, and providing a treatment plan for the next level of care. We have found that the initial time spent is an investment that pays wisely in time saved over the entire course of treatment. How this is accomplished and what additional benefits can be derived from this uniform method of treatment documentation are the subjects of Chapters 9 and 10, respectively.

Chapter 9

Progress Toward Outcome
and Effectiveness
of Treatment

"How is the patient progressing?"

The authors discuss the utility of behavioral descriptors for corroborating the patient's progress toward meeting outcome objectives at a particular level of care. In a multidisciplinary treatment setting, the initial treatment plan and the patient's progress prior to the first team planning meeting are used to organize, and are included as part of, the "transdisciplinary" treatment plan. Subsequent updates of the patient's treatment plan at regular intervals require evaluation of the patient's progress in meeting each outcome objective and a behavioral descriptor of the current severity of each impairment still being treated. Two illustrative case examples are included.

Obtaining authorization from reviewers for further treatment at more intensive levels of care is probably the most challenging, and at times vexing, component of the external review process. In our experience, when practitioners are able to focus and articulate their rationale for continuing care, using specific behavioral descriptors as benchmarks of both patient progress and continued clinical necessity for care at a particular level, this adversarial atmosphere is considerably neutralized. When requesting authorization for additional treatment services, we restate the patient outcome objectives agreed upon in the original contact with the reviewer and provide a patient behavior that communicates the patient's progress toward meeting each outcome objective. We also provide an updated treatment plan that includes adjustment of the severity ratings of the impairments in the Patient Impairment Profile. We then offer supportive behavioral statements—summarized by the impairment's current severity level—that substantiate how incapacitated or imminently dangerous the patient still may be. The "balancing" of behavioral statements that describe the patient's progress toward meeting outcome objectives with behaviors that corroborate the acuteness of the impairment provides the reviewer with the information needed to make accurate decisions regarding the clinical necessity for continued treatment at a particular level of care.

In many cases we have been able to substitute written summaries for the direct contact with reviewers and thereby significantly reduce time spent on the telephone. These reports are no more than an updated PIP, with adjusted severity ratings, the patient's outcome objectives, and descriptors of the patient's behaviors that support both the current severity of each impairment and the patient's progress toward meeting the outcome objectives. Additional details regarding the process of the treatment (e.g., what specifically transpired in each of the treatment modalities) is usually not necessary.

We have found that most reviewers not only cooperate but, in fact, appreciate the time saved using this systematic format for providing patient care update information. There are three reasons for this generally favorable response.

First, when the practitioner provides the reviewer a list of the outcome objectives in the initial communication regarding clinical necessity of treatment services, an implicit agreement is established as to what specifically the patient needs to demonstrate before being treated at a lower level of care. Second, because patient outcome objectives are stated in behavioral terms, the patient's progress can be measured, scored, and tracked by degree of improvement. We provide numerical data when we can (e.g., a 50% improvement on the Beck Depression Inventory); otherwise, we offer a subjective estimate of the patient's progress toward meeting each of his or her outcome objectives (e.g., 25%, 50%, 75%, and 100% completed). We note that the practitioner's capability and accuracy in arriving at such percentages have not been an issue. Third, in the more intensive levels of service, where some review organizations monitor the patient's treatment and progress every 2 or 3 days, evidence of a patient's progress in meeting outcome objectives for an impairment can be seen before there is a reduction in the severity rating.

Even when an impairment continues to be incapacitating (severity rating Level 3) or imminently dangerous (Level 4), the patient's response to initial treatment interventions can still be demonstrated via the outcome objectives. For example, after a week as an inpatient, Melanie W. (see case examples in preceding chapters) still required one-to-one supervision when testing her blood glucose and administering her insulin, and her dysphoric mood with alexithymia remained at severity Level 4. At the same time, she was making some progress toward her outcome objectives as demonstrated by her improved grooming and personal hygiene.

For some external review organizations, the absence of reduction in the severity of an impairment may be an "indicator" for more in-depth review of the treatment. An impairment that is not reducing in severity with initial treatment interventions is not necessarily an indictment of the practitioner or the treatment, but it may signal the need for the reviewer to learn why this is occurring. At the first level of more in-depth review, appropriate documentation and communication of the presence of behavioral progress toward meeting specific patient outcome objectives resolve the concern. If there is little or no demonstrable evidence of the patient's progress in meeting outcome objectives, however, or if the patient is becoming worse, a second-level review may be performed, which in our experience examines any one or more of the following components of the treatment plan: 1) the patient outcome objectives; 2) the treatment interventions; and 3) the PIP.

The outcome objectives initially determined for a patient may be unrealistic as the nature and extent of the patient's limitations and deficiencies are further revealed and understood in the early phases of treatment. Or, the outcome objectives selected at the beginning of treatment may have become inappropriate or irrelevant to a patient over time. In the case of Bob D. (see case examples in preceding chapters), who presented initially with delusions and acute alcohol intoxication, the PIP changed significantly in the early course of his treatment, and some of the outcome objectives determined in the initial treatment plan were no longer pertinent to his revised impairment profile and treatment plan. Lack of patient progress may also be calling attention to inappropriate or ineffectively implemented treatment interventions that would require the appropriate corrective action. At the same time, other treatment interventions (e.g., a course of electroconvulsive therapy or a trial on antidepressant medication) may require a number of days, or a short number of weeks, before their effectiveness can be demonstrated.

Patient progress may also be impeded by "adhesiveness" of the impairment (patient resistance)—perhaps due to the presence of other concomitant impairments that may be impeding the patient's participation in the treatment milieu or in following individualized treatment recommendations. In the case of Melanie W., the ongoing difficulties with regulating her diabetes and her resulting frustration and increased feeling of futility slowed the progress of treatment for her dysphoric mood. This information is helpful to reviewers who may be questioning, "Why isn't the patient getting any better?"

Multidisciplinary Treatment Planning

One of the requirements for exemption of psychiatric units from Medicare's system of prospective payment based on diagnosis-related groups (DRGs) is that each inpatient has a comprehensive treatment plan formulated by a multidisciplinary team ("Medicare Program" 1984). The Joint Commission, in the 1991 CSM, requires "individualized treatment plans" (PM.22.2) and refers to "participation of staff from appropriate disciplines" (PM.23). Both Medicare and Joint Commission guidelines identify specific elements that must be in these plans. (These have been detailed in Chapter 8 and will not be repeated here.)

At its minimum operational level, the initial multidisciplinary treatment plan is a collation and summation of all the patient assessments performed by all providers of treatment services. The CSM requires the treatment plan to include, in addition to goals and objectives, a description of "the services, activities, and programs planned for the patient and specifies the staff members assigned to work with the patient" (PM.29). While it is usually not possible for multidisciplinary treatment planning to take place at the time of admission, the CSM does require that a designated member of the treatment team develop the plan "within 72 hours following admission" (PM.22).

In today's inpatient settings, progress toward outcome has usually already begun to occur by the time the practitioner team convenes to develop the "multidisciplinary treatment plan." There is the generic utilization review axiom that states that "discharge planning begins at the time of admission"—to which we would add "and so does implementation of the treatment plan." The cost-conscious public, third-party payers, and the external review organizations that third-party payers retain expect treatment to begin at the time of admission. The team conference meeting, however, typically does not take place until the patient has already been in the hospital for 2 or 3 days.

Currently, multidisciplinary treatment plans (and/or updates) for psychiatric inpatient care usually do not reflect the treatment from time of admission. Fragments of the primary practitioner's initial treatment plan (including preliminary goals, objectives, and interventions) are often scattered among the patient history, the order sheets, and the progress notes. The documentation of the initial treatment efforts and the patient's progress during the customarily intensive first 3 days of treatment become eclipsed or overridden by the multidisciplinary treatment plan. Valuable information regarding the effectiveness of the practitioners' first interventions early in the illness, when the most dramatic changes in the PIP and the severity of the impairments are apt to occur, becomes difficult to find. Reviewers are generally sympathetic to the fact that a comprehensive assessment of the patient and the development of a meaningful multidisciplinary individualized treatment plan may require 2 or 3 days to complete. However, after a patient has spent 3 days in an acute inpatient setting, reviewers will also want an update on the patient's progress.

In a conversation with the medical director of a major third-party payer in California, we were advised that a method for daily monitoring of the clinical necessity for inpatient psychiatric services will be in place by 1995. Although some patients' clinical conditions do not fluctuate or change significantly in the first days of acute inpatient care, treatment nonetheless always begins at the time of admission, with the specification of treatment goals (the repair of the impairments), patient outcome objectives, and initial treatment interventions.

Because the medical record is still the final source of information for quality and utilization monitoring, we have designed the PIP documentation system to capture and graphically summarize the patient's clinical course and progress from the initial assessment. In this context, an updated treatment plan also describes the process of the care and the progress of the patient evolving over time. We speculate that in the not-too-distant future, external review organizations will put down the telephone and return to the treatment record—whether handwritten or computer generated—to determine clinical necessity and appropriateness of the treatment. The maxim "If it isn't documented, it didn't happen or it wasn't done" will still apply. Even now, a number of external review organizations retrospectively review a percentage of medical records to confirm information received by telephone. When all clinical disciplines organize and discuss their understanding of the patient by impairments, severity ratings, outcome objectives, and interventions, the result is an integrated and meaningful treatment planning document.

There is a current misconception that every practitioner who carries out treatment interventions for a patient must define goals and objectives for that patient. While the idea of multidisciplinary treatment planning is that the team is working together, what we have observed in treatment plans is that when each treatment modality generates its own problem list, its own goals, and its own outcome objectives for the patient, the result is "particle-ized," rather than "individualized," patient care.

In one patient's record we reviewed, after totaling the outcome objectives identified by the admitting psychiatrist, the psychiatric nurse, the social worker, the activities therapist, the substance abuse counselor, the nutritionist, the psychodramatist, and the art therapist, we discovered that the patient had 43 objectives to be met by the time of discharge! Obviously, this all makes no sense.

What does make sense to us is that at the time of initial assessment of the patient, some one person—in a hospital setting, this is usually the admitting clinician—is responsible for identifying a preliminary PIP, specifying probable patient outcome objectives for the impairments, indicating initial treatment approaches, and estimating the duration of treatment. (The estimated date of discharge, or EDD, for a patient in the hospital—also referred to as the estimated length of stay, or ELOS—is the target date for completion of the outcome objectives for the critical impairments.) The nursing staff can then develop a nursing care plan based upon the preliminary profile.

If the nurses or any other practitioners identify additional impairments during their assessments, or if they believe that any of the impairments are not accurate, their findings are brought to the multidisciplinary treatment team meeting to be discussed in the team's update of the PIP. What appeared to be, for example, an impairment of profound social withdrawal at intake may, upon further evaluation and assessment by the entire treatment team, be due to the impairments of hallucinations and paranoia.

At the initial team meeting, the first issue to be consensually decided upon is which impairments remain and which are to be deleted, changed, or added to the PIP. Second, determination must be made regarding any changes in the severity rating of each impairment. The impairments and patient outcome objectives identified in the initial treatment plan become the springboard for a discussion and decision by the treatment team as to which outcome objectives are ultimately the most appropriate for the patient in question. Each member of the treatment team may then ask, "Might any of the patient outcome objectives be facilitated by my particular treatment modality?"

For example, the admitting clinician may include dysphoric mood on an initial PIP and identify one patient outcome objective for that impairment to be "increased self-directed initiation of activities." After the team members consensually agree upon both the impairment(s) (and severity or severities) and the outcome objectives, each practitioner can specify those treatment interventions that can facilitate the patient's accomplishing the outcome objectives. The individual psychotherapist may utilize the intervention "clarify the nature and extent of the dysphoric mood" in order to help the patient identify the reasons for the isolative behaviors. The activities therapist can help the patient discover new areas of interest and support the patient in taking small steps toward exploring them. Nursing staff interventions, such as exploring with the patient the fears about being in new social situations, can facilitate the patient's accomplishing the outcome objectives as well. All three disciplines will be using their own different treatment interventions, all of which are now integrated toward helping the patient meet the outcome objectives and ultimately repair the impairment (the treatment goal). In this way, the treatment plan becomes more than the sum of its parts.

We employ the term "transdisciplinary" treatment planning to describe this process. We prefer this term because it conveys the integrative and synthesizing functions that we believe to be vital and essential to team treatment. Our method of impairment-based treatment documention is a transdisciplinary treatment plan model.

Case Examples

The treatment plan and treatment plan updates should summarily record the team's treatment efforts and the patient's response to them. The two case examples, Melanie W. and Bob D., presented below are sample formats that illustrate how the initial treatment plan, the progress of the patient, the practitioners' assessments, and their evolving understanding of the patient are recorded in the transdisciplinary treatment plan (and update) document.

Case 1: Melanie W.

Clinical Update

At the time of the first multidisciplinary team meeting, Melanie was still verbalizing active suicidal ideation daily. The day before, her second full day on the inpatient unit, she requested to be given a trial on "close observation" instead of the more scrutinizing one-to-one supervision. She was later found in the bathroom with a broken bobby pin scratching her wrist, which required two sutures. She insisted angrily that this was not a suicide attempt, however. "I was just pissed off at this place and all its stupid rules!"

At the same time, the staff had noticed that she was now showering, brushing her hair, and dressing a bit more neatly. Melanie would get herself to some of the activities planned for her if she knew ahead of time they were "easy and fun." She was unable to concentrate in her classroom work for more than 5 minutes at a time. She did not complete any of her assignments and persisted in spending as much time in her room as the staff would allow. With the staff monitoring her during glucose determinations and insulin dose administration, Melanie's blood sugars were beginning to stabilize, even though a routine dose schedule had not yet been established. Additionally, she could not yet be trusted to eat properly. Candy bar wrappers were found in her room on several occasions during the first 3 days of hospitalization.

In individual psychotherapy, Melanie was able to acknowledge that she "used to be mad" about her diabetes because it interfered with her social life. She found school "boring" and indicated that she was able to stay home much of the time because "nobody hassled me to go." When confronted in group psychotherapy that she appeared to be feeling sorry for herself, she replied angrily, "You don't know what it's like to have this [expletive] disease!"

Treatment Team Evaluation

The treatment team adjusted the severity ratings of Melanie's impairments based upon her behaviors and consensually agreed that the outcome objectives defined for her at the beginning of her care could still be met by time of discharge. Behaviors identified in the clinical update above demonstrated Melanie's beginning progress in meeting some of her outcome objectives. The bracketed percentages following each of the patient outcome objectives in the treatment plan record the team's decision of Melanie's progress toward meeting each one of them.

A psychiatric evaluation identified the presence of an endogenous component to her depression, and the recommendation was made that she be given a trial on antidepressant medication. Melanie was started on fluoxetine, 20 mg twice a day. Psychological testing revealed that Melanie was in fact a very thoughtful young woman with a capacity for introspection and insight into her difficulties. The interventions for individual psychotherapy were modified based upon that information. The team also agreed that the family would require intensive intervention if Melanie were to successfully achieve her outcome objectives. Despite her habitual truancy, she was assessed to be capable of profiting from cognitive treatment interventions.[1]

---

[1]The treatment interventions by each treatment modality selected for the various impairments are part of the complete transdisciplinary treatment plan document. However, only interventions selected to be used in individual psychotherapy are included here. Additionally, only outcome objectives to be met by the time of discharge are included here, although a comprehensive treatment plan update would include progress in the noncritical impairments as well. This allows the treatment plan to function longitudinally through the entire course of treatment in a vertically integrated mental healthcare delivery system. More will be said about this in Chapter 10.

Transdisciplinary Treatment Plan

Patient Impairment Profile   Melanie W.

	Severity	
	10/3	10/6
Critical impairments		
1. Suicidal thought/behavior	4	4
2. Dysphoric mood with alexithymia	4	4
3. Concomitant medical condition		
juvenile-type diabetes mellitus)	4	3
Noncritical impairments		
1. Inadequate health care skills	2	2
2. Family dysfunction	2	2
3. Truancy	2	2

Progress Toward Meeting Outcome Objectives

(To be met by 11/3—estimated discharge date)

Suicidal thought/behavior

1. Patient will demonstrate a 50% improvement in the SAAD Scale (rated at the time of admission) within 72 hours. [0%]
2. Patient will eliminate active suicidal thoughts/behaviors within 72 hours as demonstrated by the absence of communications (verbal or behavioral) about wanting to die. [0%]
3. Patient will eliminate active suicidal thoughts/intentions within 72 hours as evidenced by statements of no longer planning or wishing to die. [25%]
4. Patient will verbalize the precipitant(s) of suicidal thoughts/behaviors to staff and therapist. [25%]
5. Patient will verbalize to staff and therapist what alternative actions will be implemented if feeling suicidal in the future. [0%]
6. Patient will complete and present to staff and therapist a discharge plan form that includes outpatient follow-up appointments, a contingency plan of action should the suicidal ideation return, and, if applicable, the medication regimen to be followed. [0%]

Dysphoric mood with alexithymia

1. Patient will acknowledge awareness of changes in mood as demonstrated by patient reports to staff and therapist. [0%]
2. Patient will demonstrate recognition of precipitating factors for negative mood changes and seek help from a staff member or therapist accordingly. [0%]
3. Patient will demonstrate reduction in the dysphoric mood as evidenced at the time of discharge by a 50% decrease in the Hamilton Depression Rating Scale (rated at the initiation of treatment). [0%]
4. Patient's dysphoric mood will be lessened as demonstrated by staff observations of:
   a. Increased self-directed initiation of activities—within 1 week. [25%]
   b. Elimination of isolative activities—within 1 week. [25%]
   c. Increased integrating behaviors with others in the treatment setting—within 2 weeks. [25%]
   d. Verbalization of plans to be initiated with family members or friends—within 3 weeks. [0%]
   e. Pairing up with a newer patient in the treatment program and helping this patient integrate into the treatment program—within 3 weeks. [0%]
5. Patient will demonstrate a reduction in dysphoric mood as evidenced by the change from negative, self-deprecating statements to positive hopeful statements about self and life—measured by a 50% improvement on the Coopersmith Self-Esteem Inventory at discharge. [0%]
6. Patient will complete and present to staff and therapist a discharge plan form that includes outpatient follow-up appointments, a contingency plan of action should the dysphoric mood intensify, and the medication regimen to be followed. [0%]

Concomitant medical condition (juvenile-type diabetes mellitus)

1. Patient will verbalize thoughts and feelings regarding the medical condition to at least one staff member within 24 hours. [25%]
2. Patient will be aware of and understand the ramifications of the medical condition as measured by completion of a self-care worksheet that describes the condition, its etiology, prognosis, treatment regimen, and potential and possible future complications. [0%]

**Concomitant medical condition
(juvenile-type diabetes mellitus)** (continued)

3. Patient will demonstrate awareness and understanding of the medical condition by active compliance with the treatment regimen (e.g., self-initiated medication compliance, self-selected appropriate diet). [0%]
4. Patient will complete and present to staff and therapist a discharge plan form that specifies outpatient follow-up psychotherapy appointments; medical follow-up visits; names and phone numbers of physicians treating the condition; emergency phone numbers and hospital names, addresses, and phone numbers; a contingency plan of action should the medical condition worsen; and the medical treatment regimen for the condition to be followed. [0%]

Treatment Interventions

Suidical thought/behavior

Individual psychotherapy
1. [Assess the need for evaluation by specific support services: psychological testing, family therapy, social services, activities therapy.] [Completed 10/3]
2. Establish a therapeutic alliance.
3. [Assess the lethality of the suicidal thought/behavior and the need for a contained environment for the patient's safety.] [Completed 10/3]
4. Identify the precipitants for the suicidal thought/behavior.

Nursing:

Discharge planning services:

Group psychotherapy:

Dysphoric mood with alexithymia

Individual psychotherapy
1. [Identify the nature and extent of the dysphoric mood with alexithymia.] [Completed 10/6]
2. [Evaluate for treatment with psychopharmacological agents.] [Completed 10/5]
3. Encourage the patient's exploration and verbalization of the issues contributing to the dysphoric mood.
4. Help the patient identify behavioral or somatic equivalents of affective expression.

5. [New 10/6] Treat the dysphoric mood with psychopharmacological agents.
6. [New 10/6] Clarify/interpret the dynamics of the dysphoric mood.
7. [New 10/6] Help the patient develop a working vocabulary of affects.

Nursing:

Individual family therapy:

Group psychotherapy:

Recreational therapy:

Creative arts therapy:

Concomitant medical condition (juvenile-type diabetes mellitus)

Individual psychotherapy
1. [Obtain accurate medical assessment of the condition (including prognosis).] [Completed 10/5]
2. Encourage the patient's accurate understanding of the limitations and restrictions imposed by the medical illness.
3. Explore and encourage ventilation of the patient's thoughts and feelings about the medical illness.

Nursing:

Group psychotherapy:

Nutritional and dietary counseling:

Inadequate health care skills

Individual psychotherapy
1. [Identify the specific areas of inadequate health care skills.] [Completed 10/4]
2. Identify the cause of the inadequate health care skills.

Nursing:

Nutrition and diet counseling:

Family dysfunction

Individual psychotherapy
1. [Identify the nature of the family dysfunction.] [Completed 10/5]
2. Support the patient's participation in family therapy to ameliorate the family dysfunction.

Individual Family Therapy:

Multiple Family Therapy:

> **Truancy**
>
> *Individual psychotherapy*
> 1. [Identify the nature and extent of the truancy.] [Completed 10/4]
> 2. [Identify the educational impact of the truancy.] [Completed 10/6]
> 3. Identify other impairments (e.g., learning disability) contributing to the truancy.
>
> *Family therapy:*
>
> *Educational services:*

Case 2: Bob D.

Clinical Update

By the third hospital day, Bob was no longer experiencing any delusions. After three 10-mg doses of haloperidol during his first 12 hours on the inpatient unit, Bob became calm, occasionally dozed off, and reported to some staff and several peers that he was "tripping out." A urine drug screen revealed the presence of PCP, and he acknowledged that he had in fact "taken a hit of dust" an hour before the onset of his bizarre behavior prior to admission. The antipsychotic medication was subsequently discontinued. Bob detailed that he was in fact a frequent user of PCP (two to three times a week) and was drinking up to a case of beer a day. On several occasions since coming into the hospital, he stated that he felt unable to save himself from his drug abuse. While at times Bob felt anxious and restless on the unit, there were no physical signs of alcohol withdrawal thus far. Clinical assessments also revealed a conspicuous lack of ordinary problem-solving skills (e.g., how to use a telephone book). Bob was aware that he was very successful in persuading his wife or parents to balance his checkbook, make appointments for him, negotiate with creditors, renew his automobile insurance, etc. Bob was now feeling ashamed about being so inadequate in managing these activities of daily living, and he was mortified to discover that other people were aware of his inadequacies and drug and alcohol dependence also. In group psychotherapy, however, Bob also questioned whether it was accurate to be labeled as an "alcoholic" because "alcoholics are people who don't want to stop drinking."

Treatment Team Update

The team's consensus was that Bob was a highly narcissistic young man who had been able to exploit others at the expense of acquiring his own independent living skills. His painful feelings of inadequacy and vulnerability to any perceived criticism were regulated with alcohol and hallucinogens. Bob expressed some relief at no longer needing to maintain this charade in life, and he agreed to proceed with whatever treatment recommendations we had for him. Bob's difficulty in accepting observations and comments about himself and his behavior appeared like deficient frustration tolerance initially but came to be understood as the manifestation of his own negative and self-deprecating view of himself and feelings of futility about ever being able to change. While the identification of the dysphoric mood contributed to a more accurate understanding of Bob's clinical presentation—and would no doubt impact the treatment of his substance abuse—the severity of the dysphoric mood on its own was felt to be a Level 2. The team recommended that Bob continue his inpatient treatment on the chemical dependency unit, where he would be monitored with an alcohol detoxification protocol.

Transdisciplinary Treatment Plan

Patient Impairment Profile	Bob D.	
	Severity	
	9/1	9/4
Critical impairments		
1. Delusions	4	0
2. Substance abuse		
Alcohol	4	4
Hallucinogens	4	4
Noncritical impairments		
3. Deficient frustration tolerance	2	0
4. Dysphoric mood	*	2
5. Inadequate survival skills	*	2

Progress Toward Meeting Outcome Objectives

(To be met by 9/22—estimated discharge date)

Delusions

1. Patient will verbalize awareness of the delusional thinking as demonstrated by reports to staff and therapist. [100%]
2. Patient will be free of delusions for 72 hours as demonstrated by patient, staff, and therapist report. [100%]
3. Patient will verbalize the precipitant(s) of delusional thinking to staff and therapist. [100%]
4. Patient will demonstrate compliance with the medical treatment for the delusions. [100%]
5. Patient will complete and present to staff and therapist a discharge plan form that includes outpatient follow-up appointments, a contingency plan of action should the delusions recur, and, if applicable, the medication regimen to be followed. [See substance abuse outcome objective #7]

Substance abuse (alcohol, hallucinogens)

1. Patient will demonstrate understanding of the disease process of substance abuse as measured by completion of a written "Step 1" that satisfactorily records the adverse impact of the abuse on the patient's life. [0%]
2. Patient will demonstrate understanding of the disease process of substance abuse as demonstrated by a 3- to 5-page paper that addresses substance abuse as a disease, the problem of substitute-substance abuse, relapse indicators, and relapse avoidance techniques. [0%]
3. Patient will present at a 12-step meeting and/or to a newcomer in the treatment setting the adverse impact of the substance abuse and the potential hazards of substance-substitution abuse. [25%]
4. Patient will demonstrate the absence of substance abuse during treatment as evidenced by negative, random urine drug screening. [0%]
5. Patient will have at least one pass with a subsequent clean urine drug screen prior to discharge. [0%]
6. Patient will be able to specify to staff and therapist a plan of action to be implemented when there is an urge to use again. [0%]
7. Patient will maintain sobriety as demonstrated by a written personal aftercare plan that includes a minimum of one aftercare meeting, three to four outside support groups a week (including names and locations), and outpatient therapy. [0%]

8. Patient will successfully implement the written personal aftercare plan for 1 week within the current treatment setting or within 1 week prior to returning to work. [0%]
9. Patient will obtain a 12-step (interim) sponsor and introduce the sponsor to the primary therapist. [0%]

Treatment Interventions

Delusions

Individual psychotherapy
1. [Assess the need for evaluation by specific support services: psychological testing, social services, substance abuse counseling, activities therapy.] [Completed 9/1]
2. [Establish a therapeutic alliance.] [Completed 9/4]
3. [Identify the nature and etiology of the delusions.] [Completed 9/3]
4. [Rule out the presence of a concomitant medical condition as etiologic for the delusions.] [Completed 9/3]
5. [Evaluate the delusions for psychopharmacological treatment] [Completed 9/1]
6. [Treat the delusions with psychopharmacological agents.] [Completed 9/4]

Nursing:

Substance abuse (alcohol, hallucinogens)

Individual psychotherapy
1. [Identify a definitive profile of the nature and extent of the abuse, including substance abuse history and drug screening.] [Completed 9/4]
2. [New 9/4] Provide medical detoxification for substances identified.
3. [New 9/4] Help the patient identify the self-regulating functions of the alcohol and hallucinogens.
4. [New 9/4] Help the patient identify more adaptive modes of self-regulation.

Nursing:

Substance abuse counseling:

Discharge planning services:

Group psychotherapy:

Family therapy:

Multiple family therapy:

Nutritional and dietary counseling:

Recreational therapy:

Treatment Interventions (continued)

Deficient frustration tolerance

Individual psychotherapy
1. [Identify the triggers and current threshold of frustration toler-ance.] [Completed 9/3]
2. [Rule out the presence of concomitant impairments.] [Com-pleted 9/4]

Nursing:

Occupational therapy:

Recreation therapy:

Biofeedback therapy:

Family therapy:

Inadequate survival skills

Individual psychotherapy
1. [New 9/4] Identify the nature and extent of the inadequate survival skills.
2. [New 9/4] Develop the patient's awareness of the presence and impact of inadequate survival skills on the quality of his life.

Nursing:

Occupational therapy:

Family therapy:

In addition to simplifying and expediting the communica-tion of treatment information to external review organizations, the PIP system has a number of other benefits for both practi-tioners and the healthcare facilities in which they may be providing treatment services. These benefits and additional potential uses of this uniform documentation format for mental healthcare services are presented in Chapter 10.

Chapter 10

Additional Benefits of the Patient Impairment Profile System

"Based upon the information provided, your treatment services are certified."

The Patient Impairment Profile (PIP) system facilitates communication with case managers and external reviewers and saves practitioners time in documenting a patient's treatment. This system expedites reimbursement decisions and is designed to meet the newer accreditation requirements for patient care documentation and quality improvement activities. The language of impairments is also a valuable teaching tool for student practitioners. Impairment profiles can be the basis for monitoring practice patterns and developing standards of care. Impairment-based treatment documentation is a potentially rich source of aggregate data for clinical research and is particularly well suited for a computerized medical record.

In the previous chapters, we explained the benefits of the Patient Impairment Profile (PIP) system for communicating with external review and managed care organizations. In our experience, reviewers and case managers appreciate this precise, systematic way of describing patients, and they respond particularly well to the use of clear-cut severity descriptors and discrete behavioral patient outcome objectives to justify the need for treatment. We believe that the language of impairments personalizes the patient, drawing attention to all treatable patient dysfunctions and their degree of severity. Most external reviewers are also caregivers by background, and they welcome this humanistic description of patient conditions.

In addition to providing individual practitioners and transdisciplinary treatment teams with a concise, time-saving method for communicating with external review organizations, the use of the PIP system improves the quality of the clinical record and has important and timely applications for patient outcome studies, teaching, clinical research, and computerization of patient care information.

Patient Impairment Profiles and the Clinical Record

Charting in a treatment record has at least six basic purposes:

1. Communication among healthcare professionals
2. Creation of a medicolegal document
3. Accreditation
4. Quality improvement
5. Reimbursement
6. Clinical research

The PIP system is designed to enhance the quality of each of these functions, both for individual practitioners and for those in treatment settings in which multidisciplinary treatment is employed. The advantages of the PIP system in facilitating reimbursement determinations have already been demonstrated and will not be repeated here. The benefits of the PIP method for clinical research are detailed later in this chapter.

Communication Among Health Care Professionals

Unless there is consensual agreement and clarity as to the meaning of words, there is no communication. Prior to the implementation of the impairment language in one facility, we witnessed a discussion among three practitioners in a treatment planning meeting about a patient's "depression."

The first practitioner was referring to a psychodynamic explanation of the depression (i.e., repressed anger) to explain the patient's aberrant behaviors; the second was referring to the depressive behaviors that were observable in the patient; and the third was suggesting the presence of an underlying biochemical depression that might benefit from antidepressant medication. All three practitioners thought they were talking about the same problem but would have identified different patient outcome objectives based on their own particular point of view.

The first practitioner might have focused on the outcome objective of "recognition of the precipitating factors for the depression"; the second, on "the elimination of self-deprecating statements"; and the third, on "a 50% decrease in the Hamilton Depression Rating Scale." Once the impairment of dysphoric mood was agreed upon, the practitioners of the various treatment modalities could discuss and subsequently treat the same quantifiable patient phenomena. As detailed in Chapter 9, the language of impairments fosters a new level of practitioner agreement and consensual understanding of a patient's condition and, as a result, integrates a variety of therapeutic modalities to help the patient meet a single set of outcome objectives.

Legal Documentation

The PIP system is designed to provide serviceable patient care data to meet the legal requirements for a clinical record. Justifying the need for treatment, particularly if involuntary hospitalization and/or "special treatment procedures" are required, is an obvious example. If a patient is detained against his or her will for physical violence (the impairment of assaultiveness), explicit behavioral documentation is necessary to justify both the involuntary hold and the appropriate use of seclusion and/or restraints. Federal and state patient rights legislation and patient advocacy programs demand such accountability.

Accreditation

In 1988, the Joint Commission cited medical record "contingencies" in 53% of 509 psychiatric facilities surveyed; summary "recommendations for improvement" were given to another 44% of facilities surveyed. Thus, 97% of all psychiatric facilities surveyed had problems meeting medical record requirements, and these citings almost always referred to the inadequate documentation of both the treatment plan and the patient's response to treatment interventions (especially medications for nonpsychiatric conditions and therapeutic passes) (Casper 1989).

The Joint Commission surveys freestanding psychiatric hospitals and community mental health centers under the *Consolidated Standards Manual* (CSM). In acute-care hospitals that include a psychiatric program, the Joint Commission utilizes the *Accreditation Manual for Hospitals* (AMH), although psychiatric surveyors still tend to rely on the more detailed CSM scoring guidelines. For a freestanding psychiatric hospital or for an organization in which greater than 50% of the beds are designated for psychiatric and/or substance abuse patients, the physician member of the survey team is a psychiatrist. As detailed in Chapters 7–9, the PIP system provides a method of treatment documentation that meets all 1991 CSM standards.

Impairment profiles also enable the practitioner to more comfortably invite the patient and family into a discussion of the patient's needs and treatment plan. CSM Standard PM.32 requires that, "when appropriate, the patient participates in the development of his or her treatment plan, and [that] such participation is documented in the patient record." A patient can more readily discuss and relate to the impairments of social withdrawal and inadequate survival skills than to a diagnosis of chronic schizophrenia.

Quality Improvement

As part of its expansive "Agenda for Change," the Joint Commission is now mandating monitoring, evaluation, *and* continuous improvement of the quality of patient care and services provided in all accredited healthcare settings. The process, expected to be revised annually through 1994, is described in the 1992 AMH (Joint Commission 1991a). The revisions will be a part of the standards manuals for all Joint Commission accreditation programs: acute hospitals; psychiatric and substance abuse programs, including community mental health centers; long-term care facilities; ambulatory healthcare organizations; and home care providers.

Standard QA.3 in the new "Quality Assessment and Improvement" chapter of the 1992 AMH requires that there be a "planned, systematic, and ongoing process for monitoring, evaluating, and improving the quality of care and of key governance, managerial, and support activities." This process has the following characteristics:

1. Identification of important aspects of care, based on volume, risk, or tendency to produce problems for patients or staff.
2. Identification of objective, measurable indicators to monitor the quality of the important aspects of care.
3. Collection of data for each indicator, based on frequency and significance of the clinical activity being monitored.
4. Organization of data so that they can be used to readily identify quality-of-care issues.
5. Evaluation of care prompted by, at least, a) single clinical events; b) levels, patterns, or trends in care or outcomes of care at variance with predetermined acceptable care levels; c) comparison of performance with other organizations; and/or d) desire to improve care.
6. Evaluation of care, including more detailed analysis of patterns and trends and review by peers as indicated.
7. Action taken to improve care or correct problems as indicated.
8. Effectiveness of action assessed through continued monitoring of care.

9. Documentation of findings, conclusions, recommendations, actions taken, and results of actions taken.
10. Reporting of monitoring, evaluation, and improvement activities through established channels.

When the PIP method of documentation is used in the treatment record, all the elements both for effectively monitoring and evaluating the quality of patient care and service delivery and for improving the quality of clinical services are in place. The practitioners might determine that important aspects of care include, for example, the appropriateness and effectiveness of the patient's assessments and treatment interventions.

Appropriateness can be evaluated by 1) comparing the PIP with both the assessments and the proposed treatment interventions; and 2) comparing the severity ratings of the impairments with the patient's history and clinical presentation. Effectiveness can be monitored by tracking the severity levels of the impairment(s) and patient progress in meeting outcome objectives over time.

The PIP system organizes and processes treatment information to ensure that important treatment and patient outcome data are present in the patient record on an ongoing basis. This information is easily identified and retrieved, and it can thus credit the practitioners and the entire team for the effectiveness of the treatment.

Quality monitoring and evaluation activities are currently performed primarily in inpatient settings or in formalized treatment programs. However, we can expect that in the near future, health maintenance organizations (HMOs), case management companies contracted by major employers, businesses and corporations who are self-insured or offer a variety of healthcare plans to their employees, and others with a "right to know" will extend review activities beyond the usual utilization and certification for payment parameters to include quality indicators. Certainly any medical or psychiatric practice group wishing to be accredited, or any such group managed by a hospital or under contract with an HMO, will be required to participate in ongoing monitoring and evaluation activities, using either the Joint Commission model or one similar.

Practitioners have been delegated the responsibility of proving that their treatment services are

✳ Necessary
✳ Effective
✳ Appropriate
✳ Safe
✳ Acceptable to the patient
✳ Accessible

The quip "In God we trust—all others must document" applies to all healthcare practitioners in a litigious, demanding environment wherein healthcare quality has become a major public policy issue. The PIP system provides practitioners with a mechanism to concisely document the quality of treatment services.

Patient Outcome Studies

Patient outcome and patient satisfaction are receiving increased attention as important patient-oriented monitors for evaluating the quality of healthcare services. The Medical Outcomes Study is an $11.5-million project that aims to provide a patient-oriented method for evaluating healthcare based on how patients perceive the quality of their life over time. This study is currently being conducted by a team of doctors and social scientists from institutions, including the Rand Corporation, the New England Medical Center in Boston, and the University of California, Los Angeles and San Francisco. The project involves 22,462 patients who visit 523 doctors at various sites in Boston, Los Angeles, and Chicago and routinely complete 3-minute questionnaires on how they perceive the treatment of their medical condition to be progressing. This study is expected to have far-reaching effects on healthcare practices in the 1990s (Rand Corporation, unpublished data, 1989). Another interesting development in this regard is the growing number of large employer groups (each having greater than 150,000 workers and dependents) that are moving toward using clinical outcome indicators to select hospitals and physicians for their workers' care (Meyer 1990).

This emphasis on patient outcome reflects changes occurring within the Joint Commission itself. As mentioned earlier, the Joint Commission announced in 1986 its "Agenda for Change," a new project, with one of its goals being the development of an outcome-oriented monitoring and evaluation process to assist healthcare organizations in improving the quality of the care they provide. Clinical specialty Joint Commission task forces are in the process of defining valid measures of clinical performance (clinical indicators) that include both positive outcomes (e.g., the patient improved) and negative outcomes (e.g., the patient deteriorated during treatment) for obstetrics, anesthesia, cardiovascular disease, oncology, trauma, surgical care, mental healthcare, and long-term treatment (Joint Commission 1990b).

Current methods of treatment documentation reflect a traditional focus on the practitioner and the treatment interventions (i.e., "patient management"). Evaluators of healthcare services are now directing their attention to the progress and outcome of the treatment (i.e., "How is the patient managing?"). The PIP system distinctly differentiates between interventions and patient outcome objectives, drawing a clear line between what the practitioner is doing and what the patient is doing.

Clinical outcome and organizational outcome are the new buzzwords of the 1990s. Managed care organizations are now shifting their focus from cost-containment alone to the concept of "value," monitoring both efficiency and effectiveness in order to determine which treatment services may be most appropriate for a particular condition. *Managed care is no longer to be confused with managed cost.* Interstudy, a managed care research and consulting firm, has joined with a number of large insurers, managed care organizations, and powerful allies from the business world to study the relationship between benefit programs and clinical outcomes. This consortium has two main objectives: 1) "to demonstrate the commitment of purchasers and the managed care industry to the 'rigorous evaluation' of benefit programs in terms of health outcomes"; and 2) "to contribute to the general body of information linking the process and outcomes of medical care" (Meyer 1990). This group is refocusing the concept of managed care onto its historical definition—which includes such issues as access to care, continuity of care, wellness or "health maintenance," and clinical effectiveness, as well as cost containment. Interstudy predicts that "the winners will be [those managed care plans that] can deliver high quality care in an efficient manner" (Gray 1991).

Teaching Documentation Skills

The PIP system can be taught to any mental healthcare practitioner and is not dependent on a particular background or training program. It is common practice for training programs to rely on internships to teach documentation requirements and skills, and, yet, in some training programs it is still possible to undergo full professional preparation and never have one's records, although kept, reviewed for accuracy, brevity, and completeness (Grant 1981). The mental healthcare profession needs to proactively conceptualize and define what should be in a record in terms of utility. A minimum requirement includes such basics as clarity on the treatment issues to be addressed, a comprehensive treatment plan, and the systematic recording of patient outcome as a result of treatment.

The mental health profession asserted that *Diagnostic and Statistical Manual of Mental Disorders* (DSM) diagnoses were inadequate for predicting the cost of treatment for various mental disorders, and they breathed a sigh of relief when exempted from the Medicare Prospective Payment System. However, the "handwriting is on the wall" with respect to some form of prospective payment for mental healthcare, and practitioners ought to begin determining what *are* the adequate descriptors for their treatment services. Impairments meet criteria as suitable descriptors of patient conditions requiring treatment. Such a systematic way of describing patients should be taught to all mental healthcare practitioners and should be a part of their formal training programs.

Research Applications

The use of PIPs over time offers rich data for aggregate comparison studies. Some of the questions that can be answered in the future by studying treatment documentation using the PIP system include the following:

1. Do certain combinations of impairments require specific interventions in order to most effectively impact patient outcome?
2. Are certain outcomes predictable based on specific combinations of impairments?
3. Do certain combinations of impairments and severities predetermine the length of stay required for treatment to be effective?
4. Are specific patient outcome objectives predictably more achievable with certain combinations of interventions?
5. Are there specific patterns of impairment profiles that could help define different disorders?
6. Does a reduction in severity of an impairment have a direct relationship to particular treatment interventions?
7. Based on both a reduction in severity level and the patient progress in meeting outcome objectives, which treatment modalities and which of the interventions are most effective for particular impairments?
8. Does the fluidity of the treatment plan—that is, the number of changes in impairments, severities, interventions, and outcome objectives—have any statistical relevance to length of stay, clinical risk, or success in meeting objectives?
9. Does the PIP system reduce the number of denied or lost patient days? or the number of complications?
10. Is there a meaningful relationship between DSM-III-R diagnoses (American Psychiatric Association 1987) and various impairment profiles?

The PIP system provides a basis for evaluation and study of treatments and treatment programs, and it offers a better way to compare institutions. As managed care continues to refocus its attention on the quality of patient care, such comparison data will be of great value for both patients and businesses who are paying for healthcare coverage.

A number of managed care organizations and preferred provider organizations restrict access to a psychiatrist for the diagnosis and treatment of certain mental disorders. Whether these decisions, spurred by cost-saving agendas, are impacting the quality of the care being delivered can only be assessed with meaningful patient outcome data and comparison study. Good comparison outcome data can determine which level of expertise most effectively provides individual psychotherapy for a particular impairment or combination of impairments. It is our impression that debates as to which discipline is most competent, for example, to perform an assessment of a patient in crisis, conduct marital therapy, or prescribe medications, are currently fueled by concerns of territory rather than reliable research data. It may well be the case that good patient outcomes are specific to individual practitioners' particular skills and not to licenses or degrees. The development of clinical data bases using the documentation method proposed in this book will facilitate the study of patient outcomes for the different treatment modalities implemented by various mental health disciplines. *Only then* can important questions such as "Should clinical psychologists be permitted to prescribe psychotropic medications?" be meaningfully addressed.

Information Management

Of the 1.3 trillion pieces of paper used in businesses in this country, less than 5% of that important information is on computer (Novell Network, unpublished study, 1991). The opportunities for computerization in healthcare are enormous. An automated clinical record using the PIP system will be able to provide a data base for 1) clinical process and outcome management and 2) linkages with fiscal, staff performance, and risk/claims data. To this end, the authors are currently developing a rule-based software package to support the entire PIP process. In an April 30, 1991 report, the Institute of Medicine recommended that the federal government fund research and development of computer-based patient records "to improve care, permit coordination of care among providers, and lead to more and complete records" (Meyer 1990). In the 1992 AMH, the Joint Commission requires that healthcare organizations "allocate adequate resources for assessment and improvement [through] information systems and appropriate data management processes to facilitate the collection, management, and analysis of data needed for quality improvement" (QA.1.3 and QA 1.3.3).

The Medical Records Institute for Computerization of Medical Records and the Healthcare Information Management Association (formerly the American Medical Record Association) are presently drafting standard data fields and structures in an effort to develop a national consensus with regard to uniform patient care documentation as the first step toward computerization of the medical record, including all clinical information. Nonerasable optical disks promise legality and data integrity for automated clinical information systems. The PIP system is designed to comply with these recommended data fields and structures for use in both hospital and ambulatory care settings.

Conclusion

The PIP system prompts the practitioner to conceptualize patients and their treatment in behavioral terms. "Behavioral" is used in this book to describe a method of documentation and communication, not a psychology or treatment approach. Utilizing this behavioral language of treatment facilitates compliance with the newer demands being made upon practitioners to provide measurable data regarding the necessity, appropriateness, and competency of their treatment services.

This book is a survival guide in the true Darwinian meaning of the term. As competition for the healthcare dollar continues to stiffen, managed care and third-party review organizations will proliferate and intensify their scrutiny of healthcare services. A contest over who can deliver the highest quality and most cost-effective care is already under way. The practitioners "most fit" to provide convincing evidence for the "value" of their services will be the ones who survive. The PIP system offers to all mental healthcare professionals the necessary tools for meeting this challenge.

Appendix A

Patient Impairment Definitions

Altered sleep: Any disruption of the normative 24-hour sleep-wake cycle; this includes insomnia, hypersomnia, early morning awakening, night terrors.

Assaultiveness: Provoked or unprovoked verbal or physical attacks with potential or actual injury to people, to their feelings, or to property.

Compulsions: Ego alien, repetitive, stereotyped motor actions, the performance of which is insistently forced into consciousness, even though the subject does not want to perform these actions. Failure to perform the action results in increased anxiety. These actions can be trivial (e.g., checking the pilot light), be dangerous to the patient (e.g., cutting oneself), or dangerously affect the well-being of others (e.g., gambling).

Concomitant medical condition (specify the condition): Any pathophysiological disorder. Note: This includes speech, language, and hearing disorders as well as any alteration in cortical functioning (e.g., dementia).

Decreased concentration: Any subjectively perceived reduction in one's ability to direct one's thoughts or efforts or to sustain attention.

Deficient frustration tolerance: The inability to withstand normal or usual tensions arising from a build-up of instinctual demand that is not immediately relieved or gratified.

Delusions: Any beliefs that are obviously contrary to a demonstrable fact.

Dissociative states: Disturbances or alterations in the normally integrative functions of identity (multiple personality), memory (psychogenic amnesia or fugue), or consciousness (depersonalization).

Dysphoric mood: Conscious and apparent psychic suffering characterized by sadness, gloominess, despair, or despondency.

Dysphoric mood with alexithymia: Conscious and apparent psychic suffering characterized by sadness, gloominess, despair, or despondency, accompanied by the inability to connect affective experiences with thoughts. This results in an impaired ability to label affects, differentiate them into more subtle shades of meaning, and communicate these feelings to others.

Eating disorder: Gross disturbances in eating behavior, including bulimia, anorexia nervosa, and pica.

Educational performance deficit: Academic deficiency not due to truancy or learning disability, including functional illiteracy.

Egocentricity: The condition of evaluating things in terms of one's self and one's personal interests. Includes such behaviors as manipulativeness, arrogance, and empathic failures with others.

Emotional/physical trauma perpetrator: The perpetrator of committed or omitted behaviors that result in psychological or physical harm or injury. This definition includes such individuals identified as a child abuser, rapist, or spouse abuser.

Emotional/physical trauma victim: The victim of committed or omitted behaviors that result in psychological or physical harm or injury. This definition includes such individuals as abused or neglected children, rape victims, and abused parents or spouses.

Encopresis: Involuntary defecation not due to an organic defect or illness.

Enuresis: Involuntary passage of urine after the age by which control of bladder should have been attained.

Externalization and blame: The constant or inappropriate attributing of an intrapsychic function to one occurring between self and others (i.e., "I did what I did because *he, she,* or *they . . .*").

Family dysfunction: Lack of clarity and/or failure to enact the expected and appropriate rights, responsibilities, and behaviors of parents and children. This includes family systems with inadequate parents and role reversals.

Family dysfunction with substance abuse: Lack of clarity of the expected and appropriate rights, responsibilities, and behaviors of parents and children. In addition, there is continued use by a family member(s) of a mind-altering substance despite knowledge of having a persistent or recurrent social, occupational, psychological, or physical problem that is caused or exacerbated by use of that psychoactive substance.

Fire setting: The morbid impulse to set fire to things.

Gender dysphoria: Gender identity or gender role confusion or discomfort.

Grandiosity: Behavior or thinking characterized by feelings of great importance, imperviousness to consequence, excessive self-importance, or overestimation of one's self.

Hallucinations: Sensory perceptions for which there are no external stimuli.

Homicidal thought/behavior: Threats or actions by one human being to kill another.

Hopelessness: Having no expectation of a favorable outcome.

Hyperactivity: Movements and actions that are performed at a greater than normal rate of speed—as in one who is constantly restless and in motion. This includes the ego-syntonic hyperactive behaviors of children.

Inadequate healthcare skills: Deficient ability to take care of hygiene and basic personal health.

Inadequate survival skills: Deficient ability to obtain and utilize relevant survival information for problem solving that significantly compromises or endangers the quality of one's life. Patients who have inadequate social skills, make poor peer choices, or are pathologically dependent on others are included here.

Learning disability: Arithmetic, writing, reading, expressive or receptive language, or speech achievement, as measured by a standardized achievement test, that is markedly below expected level, given the person's schooling and intellectual capacity.

Lying: Making deceitful or false statements.

Manic thought/behavior: Euphoric or exquisitively irritable unstable mood, perhaps accompanied by psychomotor hyperactivity, restlessness, and agitation with an increase in number and speed of ideas, often with a grandiose quality.

Manipulativeness: Skillfullness in getting what one wants from others or being able to control or manage others in order to gain one's own ends.

Marital/relationship dysfunction: Subjectively experienced dissatisfaction in a marriage or relationship with a significant other.

Marital/relationship dysfunction with physical abuse: Subjectively experienced dissatisfaction in a marriage or relationship with a significant other involving physical harm or injury to the partner(s).

Medical risk factor: The presence of an actual or potential medical complication that is secondary to initiation of a particular treatment intervention (e.g., beginning a patient on clozapine).

Medical treatment noncompliance: Failure to follow treatment recommendations.

Mood lability: Fluctuations in mood of the manic or depressive type that go beyond normal mood shifts. They need not be biphasic fluctuations from psychomotor retardation and dysphoric mood to psychomotor agitation and mania.

Obsessions: Ideas or emotions that repetitiously and insistently force themselves into consciousness even though they are unwelcome.

Oppositionalism: Pervasive disobedience, negativism, and provocative contrariness to authority figures.

Paranoia: Delusions of grandiosity or persecution with behavior that remains congruent with and is appropriate to the delusion.

Paraphilia: Maladaptive sexual urges and/or behaviors.

Pathological grief: Unreasonable or extended bereavement following a loss.

Pathological guilt: Unreasonable feelings of guilt that do not appear to be justified by the reasons stated for the guilt.

Phobia: A morbid fear associated with morbid anxiety.

Promiscuity: Indiscriminate casual sexual encounters; a high frequency of sexual relations with a large number of partners.

Psychomotor agitation: Specific thoughts and behaviors characterized by 1) a physically and mentally painful awareness of being powerlessness to do anything about a personal matter; 2) a presentiment of an impending and almost inevitable danger; 3) a tense and physically exhausting alertness as if facing an emergency; 4) an apprehensive self-absorption that interferes with effective solution of real problems; and 5) an irresolvable doubt concerning the nature of the threat or the probability of that threat dissipating on its own.

Psychomotor retardation: Slowness of response, slowing down of thinking, and/or decrease in motor activity.

Psychotic thought and perception: Incoherence, repeated derailment or loosening of associations, marked poverty of thought, marked illogicality or peculiar ideation, and inaccurate perceptions of external reality.

Psychotic thought, perception, and behavior: Incoherence, repeated derailment or loosening of associations, marked illogicality or peculiar ideation, and inaccurate perceptions of external reality accompanied by grossly disordered behaviors, the aims of which may be dangerous or unexplainable.

Rage reactions: Spontaneous outbursts of motor activity characterized by intense violent anger or fury.

Repudiation of adult helpers: The inability or unwillingness to utilize or experience adult figures as sources of information, support, or assistance.

Running away: Impulsive or planned elopements from home without parental authorization.

School phobia: Persistent reluctance or refusal to go to school in order to stay with major attachment figures or solely to remain at home.

Self-mutilation: Maiming or injuring of one's body, including willful production of any symptom, syndrome, or disease (Munchausen syndrome).

Sexual dysfunction: Altered sexual arousal, desire, or performance.

Social withdrawal: Curtailment or cessation of verbal interaction to an extent that interferes with one's ability to function adequately.

Somatization: Organic expression of psychological disturbances.

Stealing: Repetitive violation of the rights and property of others, including taking what does not belong to oneself.

Substance abuse: Continued use of a mood-altering substance despite knowledge of having a persistent or recurrent social, occupational, psychological, or physical problem that is caused or exacerbated by the use of the psychoactive substance.

Suicidal thought/behavior: Thoughts of, or attempts at, killing oneself.

Tantrums: Dramatic outbursts of crying, kicking, and/or screaming in response to frustration. Tantrums may include yelling, foot stomping, holding the breath, striking people, throwing objects against the wall, cursing, biting, and head banging.

Truancy: Unauthorized absence from school or work.

Uncommunicativeness: The unwillingness or inability to impart information, thoughts, opinions, or feelings to others.

Work dysphoria: Discontent with the current work situation or level of academic-vocational competence obtained to date.

Appendix B

Individual Psychotherapy Interventions

Altered sleep

1. Assess the need for evaluation by specific support services.
2. Identify the nature and extent of the altered sleep.
3. Rule out the presence of a concomitant impairment responsible for the altered sleep.
4. Evaluate the patient for remediation with psychopharmacological agents.
5. Treat the patient with psychopharmacological agents.
6. Devise and implement a behavior management program for treatment of the altered sleep.

Assaultiveness

1. Assess the need for evaluation by specific support services.
2. Establish a therapeutic alliance.
3. Identify the nature and precipitants of the assaultiveness (e.g., assess whether the assaultiveness is defensive or aggressive).
4. Encourage the patient to verbalize the wish or need to assault rather than act.
5. Help the patient develop awareness of the escalators of the assaultiveness.
6. Identify alternative actions to the assaultiveness.
7. Help the patient implement alternative actions to the assaultiveness.

8. Clarify/interpret the dynamics of the assaultiveness.
9. Work through the dynamics of the assaultiveness.

Compulsions

1. Assess the need for evaluation by specific support services.
2. Establish a therapeutic alliance.
3. Identify the nature and extent of the compulsions.
4. Evaluate the compulsions for treatment with psychopharmacological agents.
5. Treat the compulsions with psychopharmacological agents.
6. Identify the internal/external triggers for the compulsions.
7. Help the patient learn to interrupt the compulsions and substitute more adaptive behaviors.
8. Clarify/interpret the dynamics of the compulsions.
9. Work through the dynamics of the compulsions.
10. Develop and implement a behavior management program to eliminate the compulsions.

Concomitant medical condition

1. Obtain an accurate assessment and appropriate medical treatment for the condition (including prognosis).
2. Encourage the patient's accurate understanding of the limitations and restrictions imposed by the medical illness.
3. Explore and encourage ventilation of the patient's thoughts and feelings about the medical illness.
4. Clarify and confront the patient's pathological use of the medical illness for secondary gain.
5. Help the patient identify nonpathological means for obtaining the secondary gains of the medical illness.
6. Encourage the patient to maximize compensatory areas of strength and competence.
7. Clarify/interpret the dynamics of the psychological impact of the medical illness.
8. Work through the dynamics of the psychological impact of the medical illness.

Decreased concentration

1. Assess the need for evaluation by specific support services.
2. Identify the nature and extent of the decreased concentration.
3. Rule out the presence of a concomitant impairment responsible for the decreased concentration.

Deficient frustration tolerance

1. Assess the need for evaluation by specific support services.
2. Establish a therapeutic alliance.
3. Identify the triggers and current threshold of the deficient frustration tolerance.
4. Rule out the presence of concomitant impairments.
5. Develop the patient's awareness and understanding of the deficient frustration tolerance.
6. Encourage translation of frustration from patient action into verbalizations about the frustration.
7. Encourage patient modification of inappropriate responses to frustration.
8. Develop and implement a behavior management program to increase the capacity for delayed gratification.

Delusions

1. Assess the need for evaluation by specific support services.
2. Establish a therapeutic alliance.
3. Identify the nature and etiology of the delusions.
4. Rule out the presence of a concomitant medical condition as etiologic for the delusions.
5. Develop the patient's awareness and understanding of the presence of the delusions.
6. Evaluate the delusions for psychopharmacological treatment.
7. Treat the delusions with psychopharmacological agents.
8. Facilitate the patient's accurate differentiation between internal and external reality.

9. Help the patient establish and utilize safe areas for discussing the delusions.
10. Clarify/interpret the dynamics of the delusions.
11. Work through the dynamics of the delusions.

Dissociative states

1. Assess the need for evaluation by specific support services.
2. Establish a therapeutic alliance.
3. Identify the nature, extent, and/or possible precipitants for the dissociative states.
4. Obtain collaborative history (from family, friends) of the nature and extent of the dissociative states.
5. Rule out the presence of a concomitant medical condition causing the dissociative states.
6. Clarify/interpret the dynamics of the dissociative states.
7. Work through the dynamics of the dissociative states.
8. Perform a narcosynthesis interview.
9. Encourage the patient's discussion with others who may have been affected by the dissociative states.

Dysphoric mood

1. Assess the need for evaluation by specific support services.
2. Establish a therapeutic alliance.
3. Identify the nature and extent of the dysphoric mood.
4. Evaluate the dysphoric mood for treatment with psychopharmacological agents.
5. Treat the dysphoric mood with psychopharmacological agents.
6. Encourage the patient's exploration and verbalization of issues contributing to the dysphoric mood.
7. Identify a plan of action the patient may initiate when the dysphoric mood intensifies.
8. Clarify/interpret the dynamics of the dysphoric mood.
9. Work through the dynamics of the dysphoric mood.
10. Help the patient develop a plan for managing a recurrence of the dysphoric mood.

Dysphoric mood with alexithymia

1. Assess the need for evaluation by specific support services.
2. Establish a therapeutic alliance.
3. Identify the nature and extent of the dysphoric mood with alexithymia.
4. Evaluate the dysphoric mood for treatment with psychopharmacological agents.
5. Treat the dysphoric mood with psychopharmacological agents.
6. Encourage the patient's exploration and verbalization of the issues contributing to the dysphoric mood.
7. Help the patient identify behavioral or somatic equivalents of affective expression.
8. Help the patient develop a vocabulary of affects (e.g., using "How Do You Feel Today?" chart).
9. Help the patient accurately label and communicate a normative range of affects.
10. Identify a plan of action the patient may initiate when the dysphoric mood intensifies.
11. Clarify/interpret the dynamics of the dysphoric mood.
12. Work through the dynamics of the dysphoric mood.
13. Develop a plan for managing a recurrence of the dysphoric mood.

Eating disorder

1. Assess the need for evaluation by specific support services.
2. Establish a therapeutic alliance.
3. Obtain medical determination of the nature, extent, and potential physical problems attendant with the eating disorder.
4. Assess the nature and extent of the eating disorder.
5. Rule out the presence of a concomitant impairment.
6. Assess the role of the family members in the eating disorder.
7. Evaluate the eating disorder for treatment with psychopharmacological agents.

8. Treat the eating disorder with psychopharmacological agents.
9. Confront and work through the denial of the presence of an eating disorder.
10. Develop the patient's awareness of the value of appropriate daily food intake.
11. Develop and implement a behavior management program for the eating disorder.
12. Clarify/interpret the dynamics of the eating disorder.
13. Work through the dynamics of the eating disorder.

Educational performance deficit

1. Assess the need for evaluation by specific support services.
2. Establish a therapeutic alliance.
3. Develop the patient's awareness of the educational performance deficit and its potential adverse impact on the quality of life.
4. Assess the nature and extent of the educational performance deficit.
5. Heighten the patient's awareness of the problem and its possible long-term impact on the quality of life.
6. Identify the performance deficits that can be remediated.
7. Support the patient's remediation of the educational deficits.

Egocentricity

1. Assess the need for evaluation by specific support services.
2. Establish a therapeutic alliance.
3. Identify the nature and extent of the egocentricity.
4. Facilitate the patient's awareness of the presence of the egocentricity.
5. Expand the patient's awareness of the impact of the egocentricity on others.
6. Clarify/interpret the dynamics of the egocentricity.
7. Work through the dynamics of the egocentricity.

8. Develop and implement a behavior management program to reduce the egocentricity.

Emotional/physical trauma perpetrator

1. Assess the need for evaluation by specific support services.
2. Establish a therapeutic alliance.
3. Identify and document the nature and extent of the emotional/physical trauma.
4. Ensure the reporting of the physical trauma perpetrator to the appropriate agencies.
5. Help the patient to work through the denial of being an emotional/physical trauma perpetrator.
6. Encourage the patient's verbalizations of anger at the victim.
7. Help the patient identify specific escalators to the emotional/physical trauma perpetrator behaviors.
8. Help the patient develop and implement a plan to ensure the safety of the victim.
9. Develop an alternative plan of action for the perpetrator to interrupt or forestall the emotional/physical trauma behaviors.
10. Clarify/interpret the dynamics of the emotional/physical trauma perpetrator behaviors.
11. Work through the dynamics of the emotional/physical trauma perpetrator behaviors.
12. Encourage the patient's participation in outside support groups.

Emotional/physical trauma victim

1. Assess the need for evaluation by specific support services.
2. Establish a therapeutic alliance.
3. Identify and document the nature and extent of the emotional/physical trauma.
4. Ensure the reporting of the emotional/physical trauma victim to the appropriate agencies.

5. Encourage ventilation of thoughts and feelings regarding being an emotional/physical trauma victim.
6. Help the patient work through the misconceptions regarding the "role of the victim."
7. Heighten the patient's awareness to precursors that lead to emotional/physical abuse behaviors.
8. Identify other impairments that may perpetuate the victim role (e.g., self-esteem deficiency).
9. Support the patient's participation in family therapy to ameliorate the emotional/physical trauma victim abuse.
10. Help the patient identify a plan for personal safety to be implemented in the event of future emotional/physical trauma threats or behaviors.
11. Encourage patient's participation in outside support groups.

Encopresis

1. Assess the need for evaluation by specific support services.
2. Establish a therapeutic alliance.
3. Identify the nature and extent of the encopresis.
4. Rule out the presence of a concomitant medical condition or other impairment.
5. Evaluate the encopresis for treatment with psychopharmacological agents.
6. Treat the encopresis with psychopharmacological agents.
7. Clarify/interpret the dynamics of the encopresis.
8. Work through the dynamics of the encopresis.
9. Develop and implement a behavior management program to treat the encopresis.

Enuresis

1. Assess the need for evaluation by specific support services.
2. Establish a therapeutic alliance.
3. Identify the nature and extent of the enuresis.
4. Rule out the presence of a concomitant medical condition or other impairment.

5. Evaluate the enuresis for treatment with psychopharmacological agents.
6. Treat the enuresis with psychopharmacological agents.
7. Clarify/interpet the dynamics of the enuresis.
8. Work through the dynamics of the enuresis.
9. Develop and implement a behavior management program to treat the enuresis.

Externalization and blame

1. Assess the need for evaluation by specific support services.
2. Establish a therapeutic alliance.
3. Identify the nature and extent of the externalization and blame.
4. Develop the patient's awareness of the presence of the externalization and blame.
5. Encourage the patient's ownership of responsibility for the issues currently resolved through externalization and blame.
6. Establish and promote the value of accurate reporting by the patient.
7. Help the patient learn to value the making of a mistake for informed action in the future.

Family dysfunction

1. Assess the need for evaluation by specific support services.
2. Establish a therapeutic alliance.
3. Identify the nature of the family dysfunction.
4. Clarify/interpret the patient's dynamics as manifested in the family dysfunction.
5. Work through the patient's dynamics as manifested in the family dysfunction.
6. Help the patient identify and develop an appropriate role within the family for each member.
7. Support the patient's participation in family therapy to ameliorate the family dysfunction.

Family dysfunction with substance abuse

1. Assess the need for evaluation by specific support services.
2. Establish a therapeutic alliance.
3. Identify the nature and extent of the family member's or members' substance abuse and its impact on the family dysfunction.
4. Clarify/interpret the patient's dynamics as manifested in the family dysfunction with the substance-abusing member(s).
5. Work through the patient's dynamics as manifested in the family dysfunction with the substance-abusing member(s).
6. Help the patient identify an appropriate role within the family for each member.
7. Encourage the patient's participation in appropriate outside support groups (e.g., Alanon, Alcoholics Anonymous).
8. Help the patient identify and modify pathological interactions with family members.

Fire setting

1. Assess the need for evaluation by specific support services.
2. Establish a therapeutic alliance.
3. Identify the nature, extent, and precipitants for the fire setting.
4. Assess the danger of the fire setting and the need for a contained environment to ensure safety of patient and others.
5. Encourage the patient to verbalize thoughts of fire setting prior to acting on them.
6. Clarify/interpret the dynamics of the fire setting.
7. Work through the dynamics of the fire setting.
8. Implement a behavior management program to eliminate the fire setting.

Gender dysphoria

1. Assess the need for evaluation by specific support services.
2. Establish a therapeutic alliance.

3. Identify the nature of the gender dysphoria.
4. Rule out any concomitant medical condition or other impairment.
5. Clarify/interpret the dynamics of the gender dysphoria.
6. Work through the dynamics of the gender dysphoria.
7. Facilitate the patient's understanding and development of accurate gender roles.
8. Facilitate an ego-syntonic gender choice.

Grandiosity

1. Assess the need for evaluation by specific support services.
2. Establish a therapeutic alliance.
3. Identify the nature of the grandiosity.
4. Confront the grandiosity.
5. Help develop the patient's awareness and understanding of the presence of the grandiosity.
6. Help the patient accurately assess personal strengths, limitations, and deficiencies.
7. Clarify/interpret the dynamics of the grandiosity.
8. Work through the dynamics of the grandiosity.

Hallucinations

1. Assess the need for evaluation by specific support services.
2. Establish a therapeutic alliance.
3. Identify the nature of the hallucinations.
4. Rule out the presence of a concomitant medical condition causing the hallucinations.
5. Evaluate the hallucinations for treatment with psychopharmacological agents.
6. Treat the hallucinations with psychopharmacological agents.
7. Help the patient identify and utilize safe areas for discussing the hallucinations.

8. Help the patient accurately differentiate between internal and external reality.
9. Clarify/interpret the dynamics of the hallucinations.
10. Work through the dynamics of the hallucinations.

Homicidal thought/behavior

1. Assess the need for evaluation by specific support services.
2. Establish a therapeutic alliance.
3. Identify the nature and extent of the homicidal thought/behavior.
4. Assess the patient for the lethality of the homicidal thought/behavior and provide a safe, contained environment when necessary.
5. Inform the patient of the obligation of the treater to inform the intended victim.
6. Help the patient differentiate between homicidal thoughts and homicidal behaviors.
7. Clarify/interpret the dynamics of the homicidal thought/behavior.
8. Work through the dynamics of the homicidal thought/behavior.

Hopelessness

1. Assess the need for evaluation by specific support services.
2. Establish a therapeutic alliance.
3. Identify the nature and extent of the hopelessness.
4. Encourage the patient's exploration and verbalization of issues contributing to the hopelessness.
5. Clarify/interpret the dynamics of the hopelessness.
6. Work through the dynamics of the hopelessness.

Hyperactivity

1. Assess the need for evaluation by specific support services.
2. Assess the patient for the presence of a primary attention-deficit disorder.

3. Establish a therapeutic alliance.
4. Rule out the presence of other impairments causing the hyperactivity.
5. Evaluate the hyperactivity for treatment with psychopharmacological agents.
6. Treat the hyperactivity with psychopharmacological agents.
7. Develop the patient's awareness of the hyperactivity.
8. Identify the internal and/or external stimuli responsible for the hyperactivity.
9. Identify and help the patient develop self-regulating behaviors to reduce the patient's hyperactivity (e.g., relaxation, imagery).

Inadequate healthcare skills

1. Assess the need for evaluation by specific support services.
2. Establish a therapeutic alliance.
3. Identify the specific areas of inadequate healthcare skills.
4. Identify the cause of the inadequate healthcare skills.
5. Rule out the presence of a concomitant medical condition or other impairment.
6. Encourage the patient's acquisition of adequate healthcare skills.
7. Identify sources of remediation for the inadequate healthcare skills.
8. Clarify/interpret the dynamics of the inadequate healthcare skills.
9. Work through the dynamics of the inadequate healthcare skills.

Inadequate survival skills

1. Assess the need for evaluation by specific support services.
2. Establish a therapeutic alliance.
3. Identify the nature and extent of the inadequate survival skills.

4. Develop the patient's awareness of the presence and impact of inadequate survival skills on the quality of life.
5. Help and support the patient in acquiring adequate survival skills.
6. Develop the patient's capacity to label problems accurately, gather information, identify options, and then evaluate the outcomes of present problem solutions for future problems.

Learning disability

1. Assess the need for evaluation by specific support services.
2. Establish a therapeutic alliance.
3. Assess the specific nature of the learning disability.
4. Develop the patient's awareness and understanding of the learning disability.
5. Encourage the patient's ventilation of reactive thoughts and feelings regarding the learning disability.
6. Help the patient identify and support the utilization of compensatory strengths.
7. Support the patient in remediating the learning disability through appropriate referral.

Lying

1. Assess the need for evaluation by specific support groups.
2. Establish a therapeutic alliance.
3. Identify the nature and extent of the lying.
4. Confront the lying, reasserting the value of accurate reporting and of one's statements matching one's actions.
5. Clarify/interpret the dynamics of the lying.
6. Work through the dynamics of the lying.
7. Develop and implement a behavior management program for the lying.
8. Monitor accurate reporting by the patient and encourage the patient's making amends to those lied to whenever possible.

Manic thought/behavior

1. Assess the need for evaluation by specific support services.
2. Establish a therapeutic alliance.
3. Identify the nature of the manic thought/behavior.
4. Rule out the presence of a concomitant medical condition.
5. Evaluate the manic thought/behavior for treatment with psychopharmacological agents.
6. Treat the manic thought/behavior with psychopharmacological agents.
7. Help the patient translate various affective experiences into words.
8. Encourage the patient's acceptance of a normative mood state.
9. Help the patient identify and utilize behavioral self-regulatory techniques for managing manic thought/behavior.
10. Clarify/interpret dynamics of the manic thought/behavior.
11. Work through the dynamics of the manic thought/behavior.

Manipulativeness

1. Assess the need for evaluation by specific support services.
2. Establish a therapeutic alliance.
3. Identify the nature and extent of the manipulativeness.
4. Facilitate the patient's awareness and understanding of the manipulativeness, including the impact it has on others.
5. Clarify/interpret the dynamics of the manipulativeness.
6. Work through the dynamics of the manipulativeness.
7. Develop and implement a behavior management program to eliminate the manipulativeness.

Marital/relationship dysfunction

1. Establish a therapeutic alliance.
2. Identify the nature and extent of the marital/relationship dysfunction.
3. Help the patient assess commitment to the marriage/relationship versus the need for separation counseling.

4. Help the patient identify and change destructive communication patterns in the marriage/relationship.
5. Encourage the patient's use of "I" statements and the verbalization of feelings.
6. Help the patient learn to practice "active listening."
7. Help the patient develop the notion of compromise as valuable and necessary.
8. Help the patient to utilize problem solving rather than criticism and blame.

Marital/relationship dysfunction with physical abuse

1. Establish a therapeutic alliance.
2. Identify the nature and extent of the marital/relationship dysfunction and physical abuse.
3. Determine the physical safety of each member in the marriage/relationship.
4. Help the patient assess commitment to the marriage/relationship versus the need for separation counseling.
5. Help the patient identify and implement methods of interrupting escalating arguments (e.g., time-outs, out-of-sight separation for a brief period of time).
6. Confront any externalization and blame for the violence.
7. Help the patient identify and change destructive communication patterns in the marriage/relationship.
8. Encourage the patient's use of "I" statements and the verbalization of feelings.
9. Help the patient learn to practice "active listening."
10. Help the patient develop the notion of compromise as valuable and necessary.
11. Help the patient to utilize problem solving rather than criticism and blame.

Medical treatment noncompliance

1. Assess the need for evaluation by specific support services.
2. Establish a therapeutic alliance.

3. Identify the reason(s) for the medical treatment noncompliance.
4. Educate the patient regarding the necessity of the medical treatment.
5. Clarify/interpret the dynamics of the medical treatment noncompliance.
6. Work through the dynamics of the medical treatment noncompliance.
7. Develop and implement a behavior modification program to reinforce medical treatment compliance.

Mood lability

1. Assess the need for evaluation by specific support services.
2. Establish a therapeutic alliance.
3. Identify the nature and precipitants of the mood lability.
4. Evaluate the mood lability for treatment with psychopharmacological agents.
5. Treat the mood lability with psychopharmacological agents.
6. Help the patient translate various affect experiences into words.
7. Encourage the patient's acceptance of the value of normative mood states.
8. Clarify/interpret the dynamics of the mood lability.
9. Work through the dynamics of the mood lability.
10. Help the patient develop self-regulation skills to normalize mood extremes.

Obsessions

1. Assess the need for evaluation by specific support services.
2. Establish a therapeutic alliance.
3. Clarify the nature and extent of the obsessions.
4. Evaluate the obsessions for treatment with psychopharmacological agents.
5. Treat the obsessions with psychopharmacological agents.

6. Help the patient identify the precipitants for the obsessions.
7. Help the patient identify ways of interrupting the obsessions and substituting more adaptive activities.
8. Help the patient develop self-regulation skills for managing or reducing the obsessions (e.g., autorelaxation).
9. Clarify/interpret the dynamics of the obsessions.
10. Work through the dynamics of the obsessions.

Oppositionalism

1. Assess the need for evaluation by specific support services.
2. Establish a therapeutic alliance.
3. Identify the nature and extent of the oppositionalism.
4. Develop the patient's awareness of the oppositionalism.
5. Clarify/interpret the dynamics of the oppositionalism.
6. Work through the dynamics of the oppositionalism.
7. Help the patient utilize discussion and compromise instead of oppositionalism.
8. Implement a behavioral management program for the oppositionalism.

Paranoia

1. Assess the need for evaluation by specific support services.
2. Establish a therapeutic alliance.
3. Identify the nature and extent of the paranoia.
4. Develop the patient's awareness of the presence of the paranoia.
5. Evaluate the paranoia for treatment with psychopharmacological agents.
6. Treat the paranoia with psychopharmacological agents.
7. Help the patient learn to "consider the alternative explanations" to paranoid ideation.
8. Support the patient's confirming or rejecting persecutory ideation through repeated "reality checks."

9. Help the patient identify and utilize safe areas for discussing paranoid thinking.

Paraphilia

1. Assess the need for evaluation by specific support services.
2. Establish a therapeutic alliance.
3. Identify the nature and extent of the paraphilia.
4. Identify any danger to specific persons and notify those who may be in danger.
5. Encourage the verbalization of paraphilic thoughts.
6. Develop the patient's awareness of the precipitants for paraphilic wishes/behaviors.
7. Help the patient develop and enforce a boundary between thought and action.
8. Help the patient identify and implement alternative plans of action to the paraphilic behavior.
9. Clarify/interpret the dynamics of the paraphilia.
10. Work through the dynamics of the paraphilia.

Pathological grief

1. Assess the need for evaluation by specific support services.
2. Establish a therapeutic alliance.
3. Identify the nature of the pathological grief.
4. Clarify/interpret the dynamics of the pathological grief.
5. Work through the unresolved grief and loss.
6. Help the patient replace unproductive grieving with more adaptive activity.

Pathological guilt

1. Assess the need for evaluation by specific support services.
2. Establish a therapeutic alliance.
3. Identify the nature and extent of the pathological guilt.
4. Facilitate the patient's accurate assessment of responsibility for the guilt.

5. Clarify/interpret the dynamics of the pathological guilt.
6. Work through the dynamics of the pathological guilt.

Phobia

1. Assess the need for evaluation by specific support services.
2. Establish a therapeutic alliance.
3. Identify the nature and extent of the phobia.
4. Evaluate the phobia for treatment with psychopharmacological agents.
5. Treat the phobia with psychopharmacological agents.
6. Help the patient identify any secondary gains from the phobia.
7. Help the patient identify alternative ways to obtain the secondary gains from the phobia.
8. Clarify/interpret the dynamics of the phobia.
9. Work through the dynamics of the phobia.
10. Develop and implement a behavior management program for the phobic thought/behavior (e.g., systematic desensitization).

Promiscuity

1. Assess the need for evaluation by specific support services.
2. Establish a therapeutic alliance.
3. Identify the nature and extent of the promiscuity.
4. Evaluate the patient for the presence of medical complications secondary to the promiscuity.
5. Rule out the presence of other impairments as explanatory for the promiscuity.
6. Educate the patient regarding the medical dangers of the promiscuity.
7. Clarify/interpret the dynamics of the promiscuity.
8. Work through the dynamics of the promiscuity.
9. Encourage the patient's reappraisal of personal values and morals with respect to the promiscuity.

Psychomotor agitation

1. Assess the need for evaluation by specific support services.
2. Establish a therapeutic alliance.
3. Identify the nature and extent of the psychomotor agitation.
4. Obtain a medical evaluation to rule out a concomitant medical condition that may be causing or contributing to the psychomotor agitation.
5. Evaluate the psychomotor agitation for treatment with psychopharmacological agents.
6. Treat the psychomotor agitation with psychopharmacological agents.
7. Help the patient identify and develop self-regulation skills for managing the psychomotor agitation (e.g., autorelaxation techniques).
8. Clarify/interpret the dynamics of the psychomotor agitation.
9. Work through the dynamics of the psychomotor agitation.
10. Help the patient formulate a plan for managing recurrence of the psychomotor agitation.

Psychomotor retardation

1. Establish a therapeutic alliance.
2. Identify the specific impairment(s) that manifests as psychomotor retardation.

Psychotic thought and perception

1. Assess the need for evaluation by specific support services.
2. Establish a therapeutic alliance.
3. Identify the nature of the psychotic thought and perception.
4. Evaluate the psychotic thought and perception for treatment with psychopharmacological agents.
5. Treat the psychotic thought and perception with psychopharmacological agents.
6. Facilitate the patient's accurate differentiation between internal and external reality.

7. Clarify/interpret the dynamics of the psychotic thought and perceptions.
8. Work through the dynamics of the psychotic thought and perception.
9. Help the patient identify and utilize safe areas for discussing psychotic thoughts and perceptions.

Psychotic thought, perception, and behavior

1. Assess the need for evaluation by specific support services.
2. Establish a therapeutic alliance.
3. Identify the nature of the psychotic thought, perception, and behavior.
4. Assess the patient for dangerousness (actual and potential) of the psychotic thought, perception, and behavior and provide a safe, contained environment when necessary.
5. Evaluate the psychotic thought, perception, and behavior for treatment with psychopharmacological agents.
6. Treat the psychotic thought, perception, and behavior with psychopharmacological agents.
7. Facilitate the patient's accurate differentiation between internal and external reality.
8. Clarify/interpret the dynamics of the psychotic thought, perception, and behavior.
9. Work through the dynamics of the psychotic thought, perception, and behavior.
10. Help the patient identify and utilize safe areas for discussing psychotic thoughts, perceptions, and behaviors.

Rage reactions

1. Assess the need for evaluation by specific support services.
2. Establish a therapeutic alliance.
3. Identify the nature and precipitants of the rage reactions.
4. Rule out the presence of a concomitant medical condition.
5. Evaluate the rage reactions for treatment with psychopharmacological agents.

6. Treat the rage reactions with psychopharmacological agents.
7. Help the patient develop awareness of the specific escalators of the rage reactions.
8. Facilitate the patient's ability to interrupt the rage reactions.
9. Help the patient develop the verbal skills to communicate distress or an impending rage reaction.
10. Help the patient identify and implement appropriate behavioral methods for rage reduction.

Repudiation of adults as helpers

1. Assess the need for evaluation by specific support services.
2. Establish a therapeutic alliance.
3. Explore the nature of the patient's inability or unwillingness to utilize adults as helpers.
4. Clarify/interpret the dynamics of the repudiation of adults as helpers.
5. Work through the dynamics of the repudiation of adults as helpers.
6. Provide a corrective helping experience with adults.
7. Encourage and praise the patient's utilization of adult figures as helpers.

Running away

1. Assess the need for evaluation by specific support services.
2. Establish a therapeutic alliance.
3. Identify the nature and extent of running away.
4. Clarify/interpret the dynamics of running away.
5. Work through the dynamics of running away.
6. Support the patient's participation in family therapy to ameliorate the running away.
7. Help the patient identify the signals of impending runaway behavior.
8. Help the patient identify and implement alternative solutions to running away.

School phobia

1. Assess the need for evaluation by specific support services.
2. Establish a therapeutic alliance.
3. Identify the nature and extent of the school avoidance.
4. Encourage the patient to ventilate feelings regarding leaving home and/or going to school.
5. Clarify/interpret the dynamics of the school phobia.
6. Work through the dynamics of the school phobia.
7. Encourage the patient's participation in family therapy to ameliorate the school phobia.
8. Develop and implement a behavior management program for the school phobia.

Self-mutilation

1. Assess the need for evaluation by specific support services.
2. Establish a therapeutic alliance.
3. Identify the nature and extent of the self-mutilation.
4. Assess the seriousness of the self-mutilation and provide a safe, contained environment when necessary.
5. Clarify/interpret the dynamics of the self-mutilation.
6. Work through the dynamics of the self-mutilation.
7. Identify the presence of other concomitant impairments.
8. Encourage the patient to ventilate the affect and ideation connected with the self-mutilation.
9. Help the patient develop alternative modes of actional discharge of the unpleasant affect states that precipitate the self-mutilation.

Sexual dysfunction

1. Assess the need for evaluation by specific support services.
2. Establish a therapeutic alliance.
3. Identify the nature and extent of the sexual dysfunction.
4. Rule out the presence of other impairments.
6. Clarify/interpret the dynamics of the sexual dysfunction.

7. Work through the dynamics of the sexual dysfunction.
8. Educate the patient regarding normative sexual functioning.
9. Provide the patient with the appropriate sexual exercises for the specific sexual dysfunction.

Social withdrawal

1. Assess the need for evaluation by specific support services.
2. Establish a therapeutic alliance.
3. Identify the nature and extent of the social withdrawal.
4. Identify the threshold of stimulation and/or the precipitants of the social withdrawal.
5. Rule out the presence of a concomitant impairment manifesting as social withdrawal.
6. Help the patient identify and work through the factors that impede normative socialization.
7. Develop and implement a behavior management program for improved socialization.
8. Help the patient identify settings outside of treatment where newly acquired social skills can be practiced and applied.

Somatization

1. Assess the need for evaluation by specific support services.
2. Establish a therapeutic alliance.
3. Identify the nature and extent of the somatization.
4. Identify other impairments that may be manifesting as somatization.
5. Obtain medical evaluation of the somatic concerns (and ensure their treatment).
6. Encourage the patient to identify and ventilate the feelings linked to the somatic complaints.
7. Encourage ventilation of feelings that underlie the somatic complaints.
8. Help the patient identify the secondary gains of the somatization.

9. Help the patient develop alternative ways of achieving those secondary gains.
10. Clarify/interpret the dynamics of the somatization.
11. Work through the dynamics of the somatization.

Stealing

1. Establish a therapeutic alliance.
2. Identify the nature and extent of the stealing.
3. Clarify/interpret the dynamics of the stealing.
4. Work through the dynamics of the stealing.
5. Confront the stealing and help the patient to recognize the value of not violating the rights and property of others.
6. Support the patient's valuing restitution to the victim whenever possible.
7. Help the patient reappraise personal and moral values regarding stealing.
8. Develop and implement a behavior management program for stealing.

Substance abuse

1. Assess the need for evaluation by specific support services.
2. Establish a therapeutic alliance.
3. Obtain a definitive history of the nature and extent of the substance abuse.
4. Implement a random urine drug screen plan.
5. Provide medical detoxification for the substance(s) identified.
6. Identify other impairments contributing to the substance abuse.
7. Help the patient identify the self-regulating functions of the substance of choice.
8. Help the patient identify more adaptive alternative modes of self-regulation.
9. Support the patient's participation in self-help or 12-step groups for continued abstinence.

10. Clarify/interpret the dynamics of the substance abuse.
11. Work through the dynamics of the substance abuse.

Suicidal thought/behavior

1. Assess the need for evaluation by specific support services.
2. Establish a therapeutic alliance.
3. Assess the lethality of the suicidal thought/behavior and the need for a contained environment for the patient's safety.
4. Identify the precipitants for the suicidal thought/behavior.
5. Help the patient develop alternative options to suicidal thought/behavior.
6. Clarify/interpret the dynamics of the suicidal thought/behavior.
7. Work through the dynamics of the suicidal thought/behavior.

Tantrums

1. Assess the need for evaluation by specific support services.
2. Establish a therapeutic alliance.
3. Identify the precipitants for the tantrums.
4. Develop and implement a behavior management program for eliminating the tantrums.
5. Help the patient communicate displeasure with words rather than with tantrums.

Truancy

1. Establish a therapeutic alliance.
2. Identify the nature and extent of the truancy.
3. Identify the educational impact of the truancy.
4. Identify other impairments (e.g., learning disability) contributing to the truancy.
5. Develop and implement a behavior management program to ensure school attendance.

6. Develop the patient's awareness and understanding of the adverse effects of the truancy.
7. Help the patient assess realistic educational/vocational potential.
8. Help the patient develop and implement appropriate goals or an educational plan.

Uncommunicativeness

1. Assess the need for evaluation by specific support services.
2. Establish a therapeutic alliance.
3. Identify the nature of the uncommunicativeness.
4. Rule out the presence of concomitant impairments responsible for the uncommunicativeness.
5. Help the patient value the right to be heard.
6. Identify and work through the factors that impede effective communication.
7. Facilitate the patient's development of verbalization skills.
8. Clarify/interpret the dynamics of the uncommunicativeness.
9. Work through the dynamics of the uncommunicativeness.

Work dysphoria

1. Identify the nature of the work dysphoria.
2. Rule out other impairments manifesting as work dysphoria.
3. Facilitate the patient's obtaining a comprehensive vocational interest, skill, and motivation assessment.
4. Help the patient assess the possibility of a job change or further education.

References

American Medical Association: Current Procedural Terminology, 1992. Chicago, IL, American Medical Association, 1991

American Psychiatric Association: Diagnostic and Statistical Manual of Mental Disorders, 3rd Edition (DSM-III). Washington, DC, American Psychiatric Association, 1980

American Psychiatric Association: Diagnostic and Statistical Manual of Mental Disorders, 3rd Edition, Revised (DSM-III-R). Washington, DC, American Psychiatric Association, 1987

Angle HV, Cone JD, Hawkins RF, et al: Computer-assisted behavioral assessment, in Behavioral Assessment: New Directions in Clinical Psychology. Edited by Cone JD, Hawkins RF. New York, Brunner/Mazel, 1977, pp 35–84

Behar D, Rapoport JL, Berg CJ, et al: Computerized tomography and neuropsychological test measures in adolescents with obsessive-compulsive disorder. Am J Psychiatry 141:363–369, 1984

Brown J: The Quality Management Professional's Study Guide. Pasadena, CA, Managed Care Consultants, 1991

Brown SL: Family interviewing as a basis for clinical management, in The Family: Evaluation and Treatment. Edited by Hofling CK, Lewis JM. New York, Brunner/Mazel, 1980, pp 122–137

Casper ES: A management system to maximize compliance with standards for medical records. Hosp Community Psychiatry 38:1191–1194, 1989

Colorado Department of Institutions, Division of Mental Health: Standards/rules and regulations for mental health centers and clinics. Denver, CO, Colorado Department of Institutions, March 1977

Darling v Charleston Community Memorial Hospital, 33 Ill 2d 326, 211 NE2d 253 (1965)

Elam v College Park Hospital, 132 Cal App 3d 322, 183 Cal Rptr 156 (1982)

Elkins R, Rapoport JL, Lipsky A: Obsessive-compulsive disorder of childhood and adolescence: a neurobiological viewpoint. Journal of the American Academy of Child Psychiatry 19:511–524, 1980

Fetter RB, Shin Y, Freeman JL, et al: Construction of diagnosis-related groups. Med Care 18(2, suppl):5–20, 1980

Flannery J, Taylor G: Toward integrating psyche and soma: psychoanalysis and neurobiology. Can J Psychiatry 26:15–23, 1981

Grant RL: The capacity of the psychiatric record to meet changing needs, in Psychiatric Records in Mental Health Care. Edited by Siegel C, Fischer SK. New York, Brunner/Mazel, 1981, pp 319–326

Gray B: The Profit Motive and Patient Care. Cambridge, MA, Harvard University Press, 1991

Grotstein JS, Solomon MF, Lang J (eds): The Borderline Patient. Hillsdale, NJ, Analytic Press, 1987

Healthcare Quality Improvement Act of 1986, PL No 99-60

Heilbrunn G: Biologic correlates of psychoanalytic concepts. J Am Psychoanal Assoc 27:597–626, 1979

Hilts P: Demands to fix U.S. health care reach a crescendo. New York Times, May 19, 1991, sec 4, pp 1, 5

Hoover CF, Insel TR: Families of origin in obsessive-compulsive disorder. J Nerv Ment Dis 172:207–215, 1984

Joint Commission on Accreditation of Healthcare Organizations: Consolidated Standards Manual, 1991, Vol 1: Standards. Oakbrook Terrace, IL, Joint Commission on Accreditation of Healthcare Organizations, 1990a

Joint Commission on Accreditation of Healthcare Organizations: Primer on Indicator Development and Application: Measuring Quality in Healthcare. Oakbrook Terrace, IL, Joint Commission on Accreditation of Healthcare Organizations, 1990b

Joint Commission on Accreditation of Healthcare Organizations: Accreditation Manual for Hospitals, 1992, Vol 1: Standards. Oakbrook Terrace, IL, Joint Commission on Accreditation of Healthcare Organizations, 1991a

Joint Commission on Accreditation of Healthcare Organizations: Accreditation Manual for Hospitals, 1992, Vol 2: Scoring Guidelines. Oakbrook Terrace, IL, Joint Commission on Accreditation of Healthcare Organizations, 1991b

Kessler K: Managed psychiatric care will continue to boom. Clinical Psychiatry News 17(9):6–7, 1989

Kiesler CA: Mental hospitals and alternative care. Am Psychol 37:349–360, 1982

Kim MJ, McFarland GK, McLane AM: Classification of Nursing Diagnoses. St Louis, MO, CV Mosby, 1984

Lyon AS, Petricelli RJ II: Medicine: An Illustrated History. New York, HN Abrams, 1978

Longabaugh R, Fowler DR, Ryback R: The problem-oriented record in quality review, program planning and clinical research. International Journal of Mental Health 6:110–121, 1983

Marmor J: Psychoanalysis, psychiatry, and systems thinking. J Am Acad Psychoanal 10:337–350, 1982

Medicare and Medicaid Patient and Program Protection Act of 1987, Amendment to Health Care Quality Improvement Act, sec 402, Pub L No 100-177

Medicare program: prospective payment for Medicare final rule. Federal Register 49(January 3):234–240, 1984

Meldman MJ, McFarland G, Johnson E: The Problem-Oriented Psychiatric Index and Treatment Plans. St Louis, MO, CV Mosby, 1976

Meyer H: Selection of providers by outcomes. American Medical News, February 9, 1990, pp 2, 38–40

Meyersburg HA, Post RM: An holistic developmental view of neural and psychological processes: a neuro-biologic-psychoanalytic integration. Br J Psychiatry 135:139–155, 1979

Othmer E, Othmer SC: The Clinical Interview Using DSM-III-R. Washington, DC, American Psychiatric Press, 1989

Parloff MB: Psychotherapy research evidence and reimbursement decisions: Bambi meets Godzilla. Am J Psychiatry 139:718–727, 1982

Peer Review Improvement Act (Tax Equity and Fiscal Responsibility Act of 1982, Title I, Subtitle C, § 2142)

POMR Project: POMR: Self-instruction for practitioners. Chicago, IL, Michael Reese Hospital and Medical Center, 1978

Ryback RS, Longabaugh R, Fowler DR (eds): The Problem-Oriented Record in Psychiatry and Health Care. New York, Grune & Stratton, 1981

Social Security Amendments of 1972, Pub L No 92-603

Social Security Amendments of 1983, Pub L No 98-21

Taylor G: The emerging field of behavioral medicine. Perspectives in Psychiatry [University of Toronto, Department of Psychiatry] 4(4):1–5, 1985

Tax Equity and Fiscal Responsibility Act of 1982, Pub L No 97-248

U.S. Department of Health and Human Services: International Classification of Diseases, 9th Revision, 2nd Edition (DHHS Publ No PHS 80-1260). Washington, DC, Department of Health and Human Services, 1980

U.S. Department of Health and Human Services: Medicare program: prospective payments for Medicare inpatient hospital services. Federal Register 48(171):39752–890, 1983

Vaillant GE, Perry JC: Personality disorders, in Comprehensive Textbook of Psychiatry-IV, 4th Edition, Vol 1. Edited by Kaplan HI, Sadock BJ. Baltimore, MD, William & Wilkins, 1985, pp 958–986

Weed LL: Medical Records, Medical Education and Patient Care. Cleveland, OH, Case Western Reserve University Press, 1969

Zimmerman M: Why are we rushing to publish DSM-IV? Arch Gen Psychiatry 45:1135–1138, 1988

Index

*Page numbers in **boldface** type indicate tables.*